Endo [barcode: MW00852598]

"My friend, Misty Marr, [...]
Lessons Learned: My Journey through Pregnancy,
Miscarriage, and Preterm Labor, sharing the raw emotions
and life lessons she has experienced through multiple
miscarriages, and preterm and difficult births. Misty
doesn't gloss over the resulting difficult questions and
anger that sought to shipwreck her faith and steal her joy,
but instead deals with them head on, providing stepping
stones of faith in the answers she found. Today I know
Misty as the joy-filled mother of many, undaunted by the
pain and difficulty life has handed her. You'll be inspired to
press on in the love of children and belief in God's goodness
as you read this account."
~ Brook Wayne, wife, mother of eight, co-founder of
Family Renewal

"I walked along with Misty for parts of this journey. The
path was uncertain at times and hopeful at others. As I
read her book I felt like we were on that road again. It
really is amazing how she has taken her readers along with
her through her sorrows and her joys. I think you will enjoy
this adventure as you travel along with Misty through her
pregnancies and birth."
~ Pam Richardson (Misty's mother)

"When the LORD allows a trial in our life, it is comforting
and strengthening to relate to someone who has walked
through that valley. When the LORD brings joyful events, it
is multiplying to relate to someone who has walked in that
emotional high. Misty takes you there on a walk to victory
no matter what the circumstances."
~ Bernadine Cantrell

LESSONS LEARNED

"In this book you will find one mother's heart bared open as she goes through her journey of the blessed gift of motherhood. Misty shares her heart openly and sometimes brutally honest about her expectations and real life experiences of her pregnancies and child birth experiences. Share through her trials and triumphs and realize that motherhood is truly the journey out of self-centeredness. A great read for anyone who desires the high calling of becoming a mother!"
~ Mrs. Martha Greene (aka "Marmee")

LESSONS LEARNED

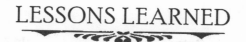

my journey through
Pregnancy,
Miscarriage,
and ## Preterm Labor

by MISTY MARR

LESSONS LEARNED

Front cover design by Perry Elisabeth Design (perryelisabethdesign.blogspot.com)

Front cover photography ©2014 A True Focus Photography (www.atruefocus.com)

Lake © Natureworks | morguefile.com
Background texture © Jaqueline | morguefile.com

Scripture taken from the New King James Version®. © 1982 by Thomas Nelson, Inc. Used by Permission. All rights reserved.

Blog excerpt © Trish Richardson. Used by permission.

ISBN-10: 0692302816   ISBN-13: 978-0692302811

Published by Marr Family Publishers
www.mistymarr.com
www.facebook.com/mylessonslearned
Printed in the United States of America

Dedication

I want to thank my husband, Nathan, who has walked this journey with me. Nathan is the unsung hero of this story. Without his support, love, and encouragement, I could not have made it through.

Nathan has carried an extra load during the challenging times. He has changed diapers, cooked food, given baths etc, etc, etc. after long days at work. And he did it all with a smile. Nathan is a true example of a servant leader, who can honestly say, "Follow me, as I follow Christ."

Nathan, I couldn't have done this without you.
I love you!

Acknowledgements

Writing this book has been the fulfillment of a long-term dream. I wrote on a small scale in my youth, and dreamed of doing more. Life circumstances brought a long break in my writing, but once the details of this book began to formulate, I knew that I wanted to go for it! I also knew that if I didn't do it now, I could procrastinate forever.

This project has also been a much more extensive process than I ever imagined it would be. I never knew just how much work went on behind the scenes when publishing a book. I finished my rough draft and naively thought I was almost done.... I have learned a lot since then! I am grateful for those around me who helped carry the load and enabled me to make this book what it is.

Thank you to Philip for being a cooperative little fellow, and a great photo companion. Much of this book was written in the early morning or late evening hours while nursing Philip.

Thanks you to Lisa Dales at www.atruefocus.com with a great photo shoot and so many good options, which made it hard to pick just one.

Thank you to Perry Elisabeth Kirkpatrick from perryelisabeth.blogspot.com for your hard work in cover design and layout, plus all your expertise in website building and all the other little details that I knew nothing about. You did an awesome job of giving my book the look I wanted, but didn't know how to do myself. You are worth your weight in gold!

LESSONS LEARNED

Thank you to Sony Elise at sonyelise.com and Alison Brace for your edit work. You guys made the final book a much better product.

Thank you to my mom, Pam Richardson, and my mother-in-law, Marty Marr, for walking through this journey with me and all the ways you have taught me and encouraged me along the way.

Thank you to all my children: Rosy, Grace, Lizzie, Andy, Bekah, Ruthie, Philip and Lil' One. Without you all, this book wouldn't be!

Thank you to Lisa Young for your friendship, support and encouragement. Thank you for all that you have taught me about healthy living and healing my body. Thank you for your time in the many desperate phone calls when I needed help in specific situations.

Thank you to Pam White for being an amazing midwife and a great support over the last few years. I look forward to going through more pregnancies together!

Contents

Chapter One

Weeping May Endure for the Night

I was a new bride, sitting in the car with my husband. We were still starry-eyed, dreaming of what the future would hold. We imagined children–lots of them.

"So, how many children do you think we could have?"

"Let's see. If I am twenty-two, and I have my first child at twenty-three ... and if I average one every two years, and have babies until I am forty-five, that will be ... um ... twelve children. OK, maybe I could have one at forty-seven. That would give us a baker's dozen!"

"Surely we can do better than that!"

"Ok, how about twenty months apart then? That would give us fifteen children. Or, if we have them all eighteen months apart, we could have seventeen children."

This scene repeated numerous times. It showed our real desire for children. I idealistically assumed that having children would come easy to me. I was strong and healthy. I never imagined that I would have any complications. Little did I know what life would hold!

One month went by, then two, then three, and I still wasn't pregnant. I shed tears each month, but otherwise I was happy. I thought the next month would be THE MONTH.

My husband, Nathan, and I lived in Mexico. My parents were missionaries, and we had lived in Mexico for ten years. Nathan had come to work with my dad. He planned on staying there six weeks, but he ended up staying six years. Two and a half years into that time, we were married. We were young and in love, and life was good.

We lived in a small mountainous Mexican village called San Juan de Los Dolores. San Juan had about 500 people, and we lived in a little house at the top of the village. The road that took us the last half mile to our home was straight up. It was so rough that it resembled the surface of the moon. Once we made it up to our home, we had a gorgeous view over the valley.

We had a two-room house which was built of block. The owners had broken out a part of the wall and had added a little lean-to bathroom. Our house was well ventilated: with holes here, and cracks there. We could watch the clouds on the bathroom floor, their image projecting through tiny nail holes in the tin roof. We even got a free shower when it rained. Our house had its quirks, but it was our home and we loved it!

We lived out in the middle of nowhere. We had electricity most of the time, and we could fill the water tank on our roof weekly. When I was home alone, I had very little contact with the outside world–no phone, no internet, no car.

I filled my mornings with cooking and cleaning, and I looked forward to the two hours a day of Christian talk radio. It broke the quiet monotony.   I spent my afternoons sewing, writing letters, crocheting, or cleaning some more. I kept my house spotless and took pride in keeping Nathan's clothes perfect. Yes, I even ironed his hankies!

The days went by slowly, but the months passed quickly. One day, I noticed some odd physical sensations, and the next day I started throwing up. I thought it must be a stomach bug, as it was way too early in the month to even think about pregnancy. But I kept throwing up. The days dragged on. The nausea kept up. I decided that it was time for Nathan to buy some pregnancy tests! Over time, I bought so many tests that I probably should have bought stock in the company.

It was killing me to wait until time to take the test, and by the time that day came around, I was confident. I had a long list of pregnancy symptoms, but I didn't feel like I could make an announcement until I had an official positive test result. I finally took the test and Nathan and I stood over it, watching the ink slide gently up the stick. First, it hit the control line, and we had one line. The ink inched up further and there it was–a second line! It was official!!! We were parents!

We quickly spread the news far and wide. This would be the first grandchild on both sides and everyone was excited. Other than being sick, tired, and still throwing up, the pregnancy seemed to be going great. I started out pretty tiny, weighing in at 103 pounds, but I quickly gained fifteen pounds. I enjoyed admiring my rounding tummy. Life felt perfect–at least as perfect as it can feel with morning sickness.

One day, there was a rain storm. I curled up on my bed with a book and a snack, planning to read the afternoon away. I heard the raindrops pattering on the tin roof of our bathroom. I jumped as the thunder boomed, and chuckled at myself for being startled. The temperature was dropping outside, and I could feel the chill. I pulled a blanket over me and kept reading. Soon, I got up to get a drink of water.

As I entered the kitchen, I realized that there was a puddle of water on the floor. I looked around to find the source of the water, but I couldn't tell where it had come from initially. I threw a towel over the water and dried the floor. I hung the towel over the back of a chair to dry. We did not have a washer or dryer, so all of our clothes had to be hand washed or carried into town to the Laundromat.

I got my drink and realized that there was still water on the floor. This time, as I went to dry it, I realized that it was in the area I had just dried. Intrigued, I looked around some more. I realized that the water was slowly seeping in through the wall at the back of our house.

Our house had a trench behind it to allow the water to flow. As the storm raged, I realized that the water was raining down faster than it could flow, and the trench had become a holding tank. It was full and the water was steadily coming into the house. I grabbed more towels, but quickly abandoned that idea. We didn't have enough towels to take care of all that water!

I grabbed my rag mop and bucket and started mopping. I soaked up the water and squeezed the mop into the bucket. I mopped some more and rung out my mop again. The water was coming in faster. I mopped, squeezed, mopped, squeezed, and mopped, squeezed. Soon, I had a full bucket. I tossed it out the door and resumed mopping. It was hard work and I was worn out, but I was grateful that I was home to take care of the problem. This continued for a couple of hours. Eventually, the rain stopped and the water slowed. Finally, I mopped up the last of the water and grabbed the towels that I had left on the table to dry up the last of any remaining water. Then I collapsed into bed. I was exhausted.

The next morning I woke up and realized that I was spotting. I was scared, but I also thought I just needed to stay down a few days and then everything would be fine. Nathan went on to church and I stayed home in bed. The spotting continued, lightly, through the morning. Nathan came home and fixed us some lunch and we ate at our bed.

At that time, we were borrowing my dad's van, which he needed the next morning, so Nathan left to deliver it. Shortly after he left, the spotting increased. Pretty soon I was bleeding enough that I realized it was probably too late. I started cramping more. I was scared and I was all alone. I curled up into a ball and cried. All I wanted was for Nathan to hold me and assure me that everything would be OK. But I knew that nothing would ever be the same again.

I didn't have to wait long. It was over so quickly. I caught the baby, so teeny tiny, in a little sac. I was stunned and shocked. I never expected that I could lose my baby. It felt like a nightmare. I wanted to wake up and realize that it was all a dream. But it wasn't.

I sobbed until I finally heard the van pulling up our road. I knew my parents would be with Nathan, as they were dropping him off and heading back to town. He had only been gone two hours and neither of us had imagined that so much would happen in so little time.

Nathan walked in the door and I rushed into his arms. He held me and we cried together. Our perfect little world didn't feel quite so perfect any more. My mom came in and sat on the bed with me, and we talked about the experience. Nathan, with tears streaming down his face, paced the bedroom singing, "Great is Thy Faithfulness." My heart swelled with love for him. On my own, I thought I couldn't bear the pain, but I knew that, together, we could get through this tragedy.

We buried our little one under a tree in our yard. We did not name our baby. I never decided if I regretted that decision, but it did set a precedent for the future. I had several names that I liked, but it was way too early to know if our baby was a boy or girl. I decided to save my names for a future baby.

The miscarriage was hard physically. Having never had a miscarriage, I had no idea what to expect. I took it easy for a few days, but the next week was a very busy week. My parents were hosting their annual Mexican Homeschool Conference, and my husband played a big role. I usually worked a lot in setup, book sales, etc. This year, I realized that I needed to leave that to others.

I always looked forward to these conferences. I knew that I would see many friends that I had not seen since the previous year. I had been especially anticipating the conference this year, as it was the first year I would be going as a married woman.

I thought back to a scene at the conference the year before. A sweet couple sat with me at the lunch break and the man began to make comments about Nathan and me. His wife shushed him with a chuckle, but he wasn't going to be shushed. He just laughed and told me that he was praying that by next year I would know that I was going to marry Nathan. Not only was I actually married to Nathan, I had been anticipating announcing my pregnancy as well.

My heart hurt at the thought of attending the conference. I was pretty sure that many people had heard that I was expecting, and there wasn't time to spread the word that I had miscarried. I was dreading the questions and necessary explanations. The joy of introducing Nathan as my husband would be marred with the news of the miscarriage.

The day to set up for the conference arrived. There was so much to be done! I had thought that I would be feeling a good bit better. I had thought I would enjoy having the extra time to visit with people, since I wasn't going to do the physical work this time. But rather than feeling better, I was feeling worse. My body still ached. I was weak and soon began running a fever.

We realized that, conference or not, we had to make an appointment with the OBGYN. I had not met with a doctor during the pregnancy, nor had I gone in after the miscarriage. In fact, this would be my first visit to an OB, ever. I was scared that they were going to need to do a D&C, and I didn't want that kind of intervention.

I was one of nine children, and Nathan was the oldest of seven. Both of our moms had chosen homebirths, and we had never considered any other option. I expected to have a midwife and figured that birth was a natural process. I never expected any complications.

I made it through the appointment. The doctor, Flor Quintana, was very kind. We were grateful to find that everything looked clear. I didn't need intervention. We assumed that the fever was unrelated, and the doctor sent me home to rest. We said goodbye to our doctor, expecting that we would never need her again. Little did we know that was just the beginning of our relationship!

Weeks went by and I didn't even have time to get anxious about not being pregnant. I was surprised to find that I conceived on my very first cycle. This time, we decided to wait a while rather than announce the pregnancy right away. That is a decision that I always regretted.

Nathan thought that if something went wrong, it would be easier if people did not know, rather than announcing a second miscarriage so soon. That thought seemed logical, and normally I am a very logical person. However, I wasn't prepared for how illogical hormones could make me feel.

Just days after we confirmed the pregnancy, I began spotting. I was crushed. I thought that the first miscarriage was a one-time thing. I no longer had that security. My dad stopped by the house unexpectedly. He had a few instructions for Nathan. He teased me good-naturedly about still being in my pajamas at 10 a.m. and went on his way.

I was angry and hurt. How could he be so insensitive? I was hurting, and he had no sympathy. Logic kicked in quickly as I realized that it was impossible for him to be sympathetic. He didn't even know. After that exchange, I realized that I would much rather have others rejoice with me with each new life and grieve with me through each death. Going through the loss of another baby without the support of my family and friends left me feeling so alone. I decided that from then on out, I would announce my pregnancies from the beginning.

This pregnancy came and went quietly. I felt disloyal to my baby. When I talked to others, I didn't want to mention that I had experienced another miscarriage. I felt I would also have to admit that I hadn't shared the news originally. I heaped unjust guilt on myself.

The next couple of months went by smoothly. Nathan and I made a trip to Georgia so that I could introduce Nathan to my family and childhood friends. People brought up the first miscarriage and spoke of the hope I had for another baby. Every time it was mentioned, my heart hurt. They didn't know that there was no more hope for the next baby. He was already gone.

A couple of months later, I felt some now-recognizable sensations. Sure enough, I was indeed pregnant again. On one side, I was thrilled. Maybe this child would be the fulfillment of a dream! I shared the news cautiously. I cringed every time someone mentioned it being my second pregnancy, and that it was normal for women to have a miscarriage. They would tell me that it usually didn't happen twice in a row. But they didn't know.

A week passed and I let down my guard. I was rejoicing in the new life I was carrying! I felt like there was light at the end of the dark tunnel. My mind switched gears from losing this little one to making plans to include him or her. I began to think about fabric to sew maternity clothes and imagined my life with a baby in my arms.

Tragically, my joy was once again short lived. This miscarriage was fast and furious. I began spotting in the evening. That night, Nathan held me as the pain and contractions wracked through my body. I was grateful to have his arms around me. I alternated between crying out in pain and sobbing on his shoulder. Soon, it was over. Nathan continued to hold me and quietly sing to me, "There is a place of quiet rest, near to the heart of God." I finally slept.

By now, we realized that there was a problem that was not going to simply resolve itself. This was the beginning of months of doctor's appointments and testing. I hated the doctor visits, yet I was intrigued.

I felt confused and hurt. Pregnancy was supposed to be a joyous time--the beginning of the joy that was to come. I felt cynical and not sure I even wanted to go through that heartbreak again. I thought, *three strikes and you're out.*

I began to learn more about my body and how it worked. I probably annoyed some of the doctors and sonogram technicians as I asked question after question about the reproductive system and the ins and outs of how my body worked together. I bought books and began learning more.

None of the doctors we saw in Mexico could find any problem. We eventually traveled to Texas to see another OBGYN--a family friend of ours. After checking me and seeing the lab work and all that went along with that, his verdict was, "I don't see any reason why you shouldn't try again." Little did we know that another little life was already forming inside of me.

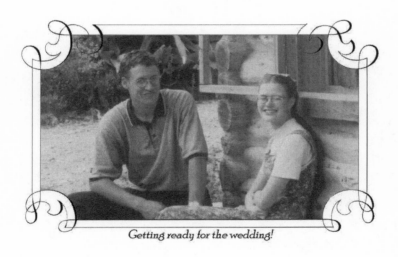

Getting ready for the wedding!

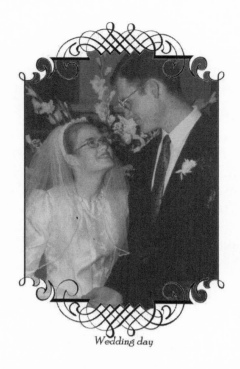

Wedding day

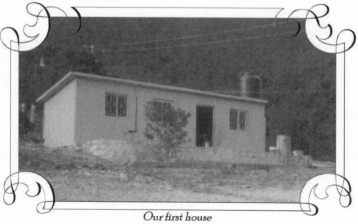

Our first house

Chapter Two

Choose You This Day

I celebrated my twenty-third birthday on the road. I had expected to have a great day, spending the whole day with Nathan. However, I ended up crying on and off. First, Nathan forgot to tell me Happy Birthday until mid-morning. Somehow, the fact that he had remembered the night before, and had even bought me a gift, didn't seem to register.

We stopped at Wendy's for lunch. We went in to eat, but wanted to be in and out quickly since we were trying to make it home that night. I asked for a cheeseburger without mayonnaise, and they forgot to leave the mayonnaise off. I sat in Wendy's and cried and cried. I was angry at myself for being so upset. I accidently knocked my catsup and splattered it on the wall. I put my head on the table and bawled.

A couple of weeks later, I found out why my hormones had been so irrational–I was pregnant! The first week after conception, my hormones were always out of control. In the previous pregnancies, I had figured that out. If I would get irrationally upset, Nathan would tease and ask me if I was pregnant. It was funny in the beginning. But by now, neither of us thought pregnancy was funny. Pregnancy was a scary thing and a setup for more pain.

Morning sickness kicked in, stronger than ever. Pretty soon, I couldn't keep anything down. Within a week I was throwing up fifteen to twenty times a day. I had always heard that being nauseated was a good sign, so I tried to rejoice that I was sick. I couldn't keep hardly any food down. The only things that even sounded edible were a few of my childhood favorites which I hadn't eaten in a long time.

The foods that I wanted were not available in Mexico. Fortunately, either my dad or Nathan made frequent trips over the border. We received our mail in McAllen, Texas, and when we picked that up, we were also able to stock up on groceries. They made the trip about once a month, sometimes more. It was a five- to six-hour drive, depending on the line to get into the United States. Sometimes we made quick trips, coming and going in one day, and other times we spent the night.

The first chance I had, I sent my grocery list with my dad—frozen pizza, canned Ravioli, canned Spaghetti-Os, Ramen Noodles, and frozen chicken pot pies. I lived on these foods for a while. I tried to eat them sparingly, but they were the only thing that I could get down—those and peanut butter hot chocolate. I melted big spoonfuls of peanut butter into my hot chocolate and ate it with a spoon. Somehow, it never occurred to me that my diet might be part of the problem.

The weeks passed, and my fear was cautiously being replaced with hope. I was still sick, and I could see my tummy rounding. The point where I had my earliest miscarriages passed, and soon I was six weeks along. After eight weeks, I felt like I was finally home free! I was really going to have this baby. I laid aside my previous fears and was sure that God was going to give me my heart's desire. I continued to throw up regularly. My days were so different than before the pregnancies. Now my life revolved around trying to get food into me.

Four pregnancies in less than a year were starting to take a toll on me physically. Before the pregnancies I was strong and capable. I knew how to work hard. I took pride in what I could accomplish. Now, I was doing good to just keep the house in order. The days of ironing my husband's hankies were long gone.

My first anniversary was fast approaching. Many girls dream of their weddings and imagine all the little details. I, however, dreamed of my first anniversary. The scenarios would change. The setting would change. But there was one thing that was always the same: I had a baby in my arms. Long before I married, I imagined sitting with my imaginary husband, together gazing in awe at the new life that God had entrusted to our care.

Now that I was married, my first anniversary dreams didn't fade. I had come to terms with the fact that I would not be holding my baby in my arms. I carried my baby inside, and I could accept that. As the big day approached, my daydreams increased. I re-created all my earlier scenarios, making them work with my being pregnant. I couldn't wait to celebrate one year of marriage to Nathan and the new life I was holding. Once again, life started to feel perfect.

One day, two months into the pregnancy, I woke up in the early morning hour. Our well-ventilated house was chilly. The tile floor felt icy, and I could feel the breeze coming through the cracks in the bathroom. I wanted to get back to my bed and under my quilt, which I had made from the scraps of many of my old dresses.

I felt a pop and instantly knew something was wrong. In horror, I watched as the toilet filled with blood–blood necessary for the life of my baby. The blood was gushing and I quickly went from fearing not only for the life of my baby, but for mine as well. I had heard stories of women hemorrhaging, but I never expected it to happen to me. As quickly as the bleeding started, it stopped. I stumbled back to my bed in shock.

Nathan held me and prayed that God would spare the life of our baby, though I felt it was too late. We knew that I should go into the hospital, but we were not sure that I could make the trip. The closest hospital to us was two hours away, in the city of Saltillo, Mexico. The bumpy dirt roads leading to our house made an arduous drive and could leave our teeth rattling. Because of the amount of blood that I had just lost, we felt that the bumping and jostling of the trip could trigger the hemorrhage and be a bigger threat than staying put. So we waited.

I continued to bleed throughout the day, but it lightened up by the next day. My heart couldn't handle another letdown, so I continued to insist that it was too late. The days of bed rest dragged on and the bleeding got lighter and lighter, but we weren't confident that I had actually passed the baby. I started to get a glimmer of hope as the blood let up to almost nothing

The week passed slowly, the hours inching by. I tossed in my bed restlessly, wondering and waiting. I couldn't let myself hope, yet I couldn't give up hope entirely. Each day seemed like it was that much safer for me to make the trip to the doctor. We decided that Monday was the day. I was relieved to have a date. Not knowing felt harder than just dealing with the grief. I was ready for answers!

Saturday night, I felt another pop. "Not again!" I exclaimed. But it was true. I was hemorrhaging again. The bleeding was less and didn't last as long as it had the previous week, but it seemed to confirm that I had indeed lost this baby.

We woke up Sunday morning to a dreary, damp day. I was no longer bleeding and it seemed safe for me to be alone, so Nathan headed out to pick up people for church. I stayed home, chilled and alone. It was my first anniversary.

I tried to hold all my emotions in, but once Nathan was gone, I let loose. I began to cry out to God, with my heart full of anger and hurt.

"Why, God? Why are You doing this to me again? You promised that if I delighted in You, You would give me the desire of my heart. I have followed You. I spent my youth serving You. I've sacrificed so much, and I have done it cheerfully, truly happy to please You. You tested me by taking my baby, and I still trusted You. And You did it again and again. And now You are taking my fourth baby? You are putting me through this again. On the one day I most dreamed of holding my baby, You are ripping it away from me. If this is how You repay all I have done for You, I don't know if I even want to serve You."

I finally spoke the words that I had been unwilling to acknowledge. I lashed out at God, pouring out the feelings I had been holding back, and I broke down weeping. I sobbed for two hours. I didn't want to stop crying. I knew that once I settled down, I would have to think. I didn't want to think about how I felt. I knew that I couldn't just move on and let things go back to normal. I had to face my feelings and deal with them. I had to make a decision.

My tears finally subsided and I wearily fell into a restless sleep. Tossing and turning, not even my dreams would let me escape my flurry of emotions. I woke more exhausted than I had been, my previously smooth blanket, now rumpled and twisted. The weight of the words I had spoken hit me like a ton of bricks. I sank back into the bed and pulled the blanket up to my chin, finally allowing myself to think.

I felt as though this was a test and God was setting out an ultimatum. Would I trust Him, no matter what, or would I reject Him and turn away? As I thought back through my life, all my memories revolved around serving the Lord. Pleasing God had been my mantra and the driving force behind all my decisions. Could I just lay that aside and walk away? Who was I without God? What would be left of me if I walked away?

I thought back to learning about God as a child. I thought through all I had done for Him as a youth. I analyzed all that I had sacrificed for His sake. Then I began to compare it to what He had done for me, what He had sacrificed for me, and all that He had given to me. It began to dawn on me that all my righteousness truly was like filthy rags in comparison.

I thought of all the hard times and struggles when God was at my side, carrying me through. We had so many stories of needs that God had provided. There was so much good and so much joy in my life, and that all had come from God.

I remembered the verse in James that says that every good and perfect gift comes from above. Next, I thought of the verse that said, "Though He slay me, yet I will trust Him." And, finally, "All things work together for good to them that love the Lord" came through my mind. I realized that even in the midst of my anger, God was still faithful to bring His words to my mind-just the ones that I needed to hear.

I realized that in light of the evidence of who God was, and the reality of who I was, I had no choice. I had to choose to trust, no matter what God asked of me. I decided that I would say, as Job said, "The Lord has given and the Lord has taken away. Blessed be the name of the Lord."

I prayed and cried again, and once again I fell asleep. This time my sleep was not fitful; it was untroubled and gave rest to my weary soul.

Monday morning dawned bright and cheery. I anxiously got up and ready to head out to the city for our doctor's appointment. My biggest concern was that they would say that I hadn't passed everything and would need a D&C. The car bumped along the dirt road, but didn't cause anything more than a little discomfort. We arrived and my stomach felt sick as we waited our turn. I dreaded the news, assuming that we would have the final confirmation of our baby's death.

Dr. Flor Quintana was kind and understanding. Nathan held my hand as she prepared the sonogram probe and squirted the gel on my tummy. We had our eyes glued to the monitor. It took a split second to register what we were seeing.

"Your baby is very active and definitely alive," Dr. Quintana announced.

Soon, we had a diagnosis and cause for the hemorrhaging: placenta previa. The gushes of blood had come from the placenta, and as long as we kept that from happening again, our baby would be fine! The doctor prescribed bed rest, and assured us that there was a good chance of the placenta moving up on its own.

We went back to the car and I cried again-this time with tears of joy! I had hope once again. My baby was actually alive.

The next couple of months dragged on slowly. I was home alone most days. Nathan would make sure I had everything I needed beside my bed in the mornings, before he headed out to work on whatever project my dad had for him. Every few weeks, we headed back to town for another appointment, and each one showed that my placenta was moving up in the right direction.

Finally the big day came and the doctor announced that we were going to have a girl! We named our daughter Rosanna Joy. I chose the name Rosanna when I was seven years old, and Joy fit so well since we were so full of joy to finally have a baby!

When my next doctor appointment arrived, the sonogram showed that my placenta had moved up and was no longer covering the cervical opening! We were ecstatic. Not only did this mean that I would be safe for a natural birth, rather than a C-Section, it also meant that I was no longer high risk and I could get off bed rest.

We went out to eat in town to celebrate before we returned home. I felt like I could finally be a normal pregnant woman. Since I had been on bed rest for so long, I knew I had my work cut out for me. My house desperately needed my attention!

At home, I began the process of cleaning and organizing. Our house was small. We just had two rooms--the kitchen and our bedroom--and the square footage was less than 500 square feet. Some argued that a house that small was so much easier to clean, but the other side of the coin was that we didn't have much storage space. There were no closets in the house and we only had one small countertop with cabinets in the kitchen. We had purchased a small cabinet to hang our clothes in, but much of our clothes and other belongings were stored in cardboard boxes.

I kept my eyes out for sturdy boxes, and stacked them with the tops facing out, so I was able to use them like shelves. I spent the next few weeks cleaning, organizing, and enjoying being pregnant. My house was finally getting back in shape. My baby was healthy and active. I thought we had finally left behind the pregnancy complications and could now return to a normal life.

Now that the pregnancy was no longer high risk, we were able to make our appointments with the doctor who would deliver Rosy at home--Irma. We couldn't imagine any option other than home birth. Nathan and I both had a lot of younger siblings, and both of our moms had chosen home births. Home births were a given in our mind.

Because our house was so far out of town, we compromised and decided to have our birth at the house in the small town of Arteaga. I used to live in this house with my parents, but it was now being used as the ministry office. Most of the house was still set up as we left it, with the bedrooms and kitchen still very homey. We spent a lot time there already, when Nathan had ministry projects to work on.

One day I felt a twinge. What was that? I asked around and the moms around me said that it was just a Braxton Hicks contraction and was nothing to worry about. I'd heard of Braxton Hicks and since I didn't have anything to compare them with, I assumed they were right. Over the next few days, the feelings increased in intensity and in quantity.

I held my hand over my rock-hard tummy, doubled over in pain. *This doesn't feel right,* I thought. I found that any activity increased the contractions. I thought that all women had Braxton Hicks, and I had known lots of pregnant women, but I had never seen a pregnant woman act like they felt what I was feeling. At first I thought I was just a wimp. Maybe I was overly cautious because of my miscarriage experiences.

Finally, at twenty-eight weeks, I knew something was wrong. We went back to our doctor. She checked me and had another sonogram. "Is it still a girl?" Nathan quipped. She confirmed that our baby was a girl, and she was healthy, active and growing perfectly. The Dr Flor Quintana diagnosed me with preterm labor.

My heart sank with the news of preterm labor. "How many things can go wrong?" I wondered. "Will I lose my baby after all this?" I felt sick, but Dr. Quintana assured me that if I followed her instructions, everything should be OK.

The first instruction was more bed rest. She also prescribed medication to stop the contractions. I went home and back to bed. Again. Little did I know that my experience with bed rest was just beginning!

I had Nathan gather up the leftover fabric from my favorite dress and my sewing supplies. I measured and cut and stitched. A little dress with pink flowers began to form. I felt like Laura Ingalls Wilder, hand stitching my little baby dress. I might not be able to get up and sew, but I could stitch in bed. I cut up a rose-colored sheet for the contrast and added ruffles and bows.

I had sewn most of my clothes, but I was determined that this little dress would be my best. I would not have imagined that ten years and five daughters later, the dress would still be going strong.

The days dragged by. I was glad that I had the chance to catch up on the house before this period of bed rest started, but I was losing ground quickly. I would lie in the empty house, looking around at all the things I wanted to do, but couldn't. Nathan would fix us both breakfast, make sure there was food out for me for lunch, and head out to work. He got home in time to fix us supper.

Most days I was completely alone. Without a phone or computer, I had no contact with the outside world, apart from one small Christian radio station that we could pick up all the way down there in Mexico. Talk radio played from noon till 2:00 p.m., and I looked forward to listening to Family Life Today and Focus on the Family every day.

I spent a lot of my time reading about natural birth. I especially loved one of the books that talked about relaxation and birth without pain. I reread that book over and over. I was sure that I had a good grasp of the techniques taught and that I would be able to sail through this labor. Sure, I knew that there would be *some* pain. I mean, really, a baby coming out HAS to hurt! It wouldn't be called labor if it weren't hard work. But I felt like I would be able to stay in control and that I would be stronger than the labor. I knew I would go into labor with confidence.

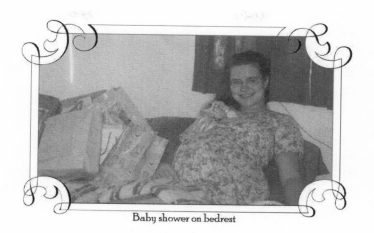

Baby shower on bedrest

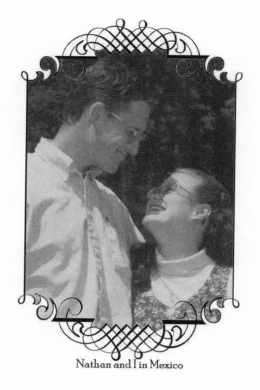

Nathan and I in Mexico

Chapter Three

Struggling to Progress

Finally, week thirty-six came and it was time to stop the medication. I had been taking the pill every eight hours. About six to seven hours after each dose, my contractions would pick up. I would take the medication and they would let back up. I suspected that once I got the medication out of my system, labor would come quickly.

I took my last pill on Sunday night and then I got up for the first time in weeks and started packing our bags. I had a number of contractions before we drove out to Arteaga, where we planned to stay until after the birth. Because of the extra exertion, I was tired and slept soundly.

I woke up with a start on Monday morning. "Wow, that was some contraction," I thought. "It's the strongest one I've had yet." Soon there was another and then another. I pulled out my watch and started timing them. I finally woke Nathan up and told him that I thought it was time.

We got up and I puttered around the house, trying to get things unpacked and pulled out my birth kit. We lined the bed with a plastic sheet and laid out everything we would need.

Contractions increased slowly, but consistently. We let my mom know that it was time and called Dr. Irma. When Irma checked me, she confirmed that this was the real thing. I was excited to get with it! Going to bed that night with a wee baby in my arms sounded like heaven on earth.

I smoothed out the little pink blankets in my cradle. Rosy's bed had been a gift to my mom when she was expecting me! My mom worked hard sanding each rung, and my dad stained and varnished it. Things had come full circle. First I slept in it, and then it was my doll bed. Next, all my little siblings used it. It was finally time for my baby! I sorted through the little clothes and lovingly laid out her first outfit.

The doctor told Nathan that walking would really help me, and he took that to heart. He took me outside to the back patio and we walked in circles around it. We walked and walked and walked! We stopped every few minutes, so I could hold onto Nathan's neck and breathe through each contraction. And then we kept walking. I was getting exhausted. I had been on bed rest so much of this pregnancy, my body was not used to this kind of exertion. But we were sure that it was the best thing for me and the labor, so we pressed through!

We came inside and I collapsed into the recliner. My mom asked me what I wanted to eat. "I will make you whatever you want," she told me. And then she quipped,

"It looks like roles have reversed!" My mom had me and eight other children, but six of my siblings were ages nine and under! I had made my mom her labor cravings many times.

I knew exactly what I wanted for lunch--chicken soup. I wanted the real stuff: homemade, lots of broth, seasoned with garlic, and plenty of veggies. I reclined and timed contractions while the scent of the soup cooking wafted through the air. Contractions were picking up, the soup smelled delicious, and this labor was going perfectly. Ever since that day, chicken soup makes me feel so content and satisfied. It is my biggest craving during labor and after birth.

My mom and Doctor Irma sat and visited. Since Doctor Irma had small children, she was not currently practicing, except for a few patients in her home. She had delivered several of my siblings, so my mom enjoyed being on the other side of things this time.

After lunch, Doctor Irma checked me: five centimeters and things were progressing nicely. Nathan took me back out to walk. I was stopping more often and the contractions were getting longer. We would get halfway around the circle and another contraction would come. And another and another. Pretty soon those contractions were on top of each other.

She checked me again and we were at seven centimeters and then nine. "It will be very soon now," they assured me. We headed to the bedroom for the final leg of labor. Or so we thought.

The contractions intensified and, suddenly, I no longer felt in control. I was somehow comforted by that thought, because everything I had read said that was a natural response to transition and that it was almost time. I was finally given the go-ahead to push.

The excitement of knowing that Rosy was almost out gave me strength. I pushed with renewed vigor. "I can feel her head," Doctor Irma announced. It was Sunday evening. Twelve hours of labor and we were in the home stretch. Or so I thought.

I began to push, giving it all I could. The excitement of being so close to holding my baby was bigger than the pain. I knew that some people had their babies with just a few pushes, but since this was my first baby, I knew it could be much longer. I had mentally prepared myself for an hour of pushing, though hoping to cut that at least in half.

I remained in control that first hour. The contractions came hard and I pushed strong. I relished the space between them, too. I focused on breathing and relaxing between every contraction, and that helped renew my strength for the next one.

But that hour came and went. Another hour inched by, and then the third hour was gone. They were starting to get concerned that Rosy wasn't coming and checked me again. She had me push a few more times, while feeling for Rosy's head. It was down low and seemed to be in the right position for imminent birth. It came down lower when I pushed, but then stopped short of birth.

An internal exam showed that there was a little lip on my cervix, and she thought maybe that was preventing Rosy from coming the rest of the way down. She began to hold it back while I pushed. The pain took on a whole new level of intensity. But the pain didn't pay off. We continued this contraction after contraction, with no success. I was done.

Four hours of pushing had gone by--sixteen hours of labor. I looked out the window to see the sun going down. Dr. Irma suggested that I take a break. The contractions continued to come every few minutes, but I had no strength left to push.

The rest of the night went by in a blur. The contractions kept coming consistently. We rotated between pushing for a while and resting. Dr. Irma kept a close watch on Rosy's heartbeat. She asked if I wanted to go in to the hospital, but I balked. She told me that she would take me in at the first indication that Rosy was struggling, but that as long as she was doing well, she would let me stay home.

Rosy's heartbeat stayed strong and steady. I had hoped that each contraction would be the one that would bring her the rest of the way down. Her head almost crowned with each push, but not quite.

The sun rose, casting light through the window. I had never expected a twenty-four-hour labor. The day went by in a blur. I continued to have consistent transition contractions. I would push for an hour, and then just endure the contractions for a few hours. We repeated that cycle the entire day.

Nathan suggested we try walking again to see if that would help. I refused! My mom went out for some castor oil. That always brought her babies on, and she was sure that it was just what I needed. The smell of the castor oil turned my stomach, and it came up just as fast as it went down. My mom poured out another spoonful of the thick odious oil, but this time the gag reflex set in before I could even get it to my mouth. Gagging on top of contractions didn't work for me. I pushed the oil away, and said, "No more."

I sat in the chair with my head in my hands, watching my mom, Nathan, and Dr. Irma talk in hushed tones. They decided that I should try to go to bed, but that I couldn't hold out much longer at home. Irma kept checking Rosy's heart through the night. She was holding out strong, but I was not.

I dozed between contractions, but didn't sleep much. Fears of going to the hospital raced through my mind. I didn't want to go. I had previously been leery of the unnecessary intervention, but now my biggest fear was having a C-Section. I wanted to go on to have a large family, and having a C-Section with my first would really complicate things. I was determined to stay strong as long as I could.

Wednesday morning dawned and Irma announced that she couldn't stay at my house. She needed to get back to her family, but she couldn't leave me either. She gave me two options. I could either go be admitted to the hospital now, or she could take me in to get a sonogram to see if we could figure out what was preventing birth. Irma said that if the sonogram went well, she could take me to her house to give birth there.

When Dr. Flor Quintana did my sonogram and checked me, she said, "What are you doing here? This baby will be born in twenty minutes. If you don't want to have the baby in the car, you'd better hurry." She said the baby looked great, and everything was fine with me. She clearly did not believe that I had been in labor over fifty hours!

Irma took me to her home. After she got a room all set up for me, she decided to take me to her office and break my water. I would have normally been opposed to that level of intervention, but at this point, I was open to anything that would encourage Rosy to be born.

Unfortunately, because Rosy was so low and the bag so tight against her head, Irma couldn't break the water. She tried multiple times, but it just wouldn't work. They discussed Pitocin, but decided against it. My problem clearly was not lack of contractions. I had experienced steady contractions for three days now, and had been fully dilated most of that time.

That night and the next day continued on with no changes. On Friday, Irma was more proactive in trying to help me complete birth. We tried different positions and a variety of different birthing techniques. The details of those two days are foggy. By this point I was utterly exhausted. I had eaten, drank and slept very little since Monday morning.

Finally, my body said "enough" and I went into shock. Everything went hazy. My body was thrashing around, and the pain level went through the roof. I didn't know what was happening to me, I just knew that something was wrong. The people around me suddenly felt like they were part of the background and I was drifting away. I was confused. Irma had been shouting, "Push, Misty! Push!" but now she seemed so far away. And I was done with pushing.

For the first time in five days, I felt my body relax. I decided that I must be dying. I thought that when I was gone, they would rush me to the hospital to save Rosy. I asked Nathan to take good care of her. I had a twinge of regret about not meeting her after all that, but then I just felt peace. I was ready to go. I drifted in and out of consciousness.

Nathan, my mom and Irma rushed around to take me to the hospital. Then, all of a sudden they realized that I had just fallen asleep. They checked my vitals and everything looked good. They checked Rosy and her heart sounded good too. Because I had only slept a few hours in all this time, they decided to let me sleep. I slept soundly for two hours. It was my first break from contractions since Monday.

I opened my eyes, struggling to figure out where I was and what was happening. Then a contraction hit and I remembered. *"I guess I didn't die after all,"* I thought. As soon as I started to stir, Nathan kissed me and told me that we were going to the hospital. I started to protest, thinking that the sleep had given me enough strength to finish labor, but Nathan said no, I was going now. It was no longer up to me.

They called Dr. Quintana and told her we were coming in. She laughed, thinking it was a joke. She had given me twenty minutes, three days ago. She sobered up quickly when Irma assured her that it was not a joke, and she started prepping things for a possible C-Section.

When I arrived, the hospital had a whole team waiting for me. I had always insisted that I would never allow a male doctor to deliver my baby or any male, except my husband, to be in the delivery room. Rosy was going to be born in a roomful of both men and women. By this point, I didn't even care.

Dr. Quintana checked Rosy and me, and immediately hooked me up to IVs. She said that, besides severe dehydration, everything looked fine. She couldn't see any reason why Rosy hadn't come yet. She knew how opposed I was to a C-Section, so she agreed to give me two hours. If Rosy wasn't born in that time, I would have no choice.

She gave me an IV of Pitocin and brought in an anesthesiologist to numb me just enough to take the edge off the pain. Then she was finally able to successfully break my water. I continued to have transition contractions the entire time they prepped me, and then the action began. I had one man standing over me, using both arms to push the top of my stomach, during the contractions, while Dr. Quintana manipulated Rosy's head.

There was a lot of confusion, yelling, and pain. But the sleep had refreshed me, the IV seemed to renew my strength, and I was able to go on an adrenaline rush. They yelled for me to push while the man pushed on my stomach with all his weight, and Dr. Quintana gave me an episiotomy. Thus Rosy was born!

Before I could process the fact that she was born, they held Rosy up for one quick kiss and whisked her off. They came back a few minutes later to tell us that she weighed five pounds, twelve ounces, and that she looked perfect. They informed me that they would be keeping her for two hours for observation. I nodded numbly, too exhausted to protest. They stitched me up and wheeled me to my room. I shut my eyes and was asleep within seconds.

I awoke to a knock on my door. "I'm bringing you your baby," the nurse announced. "She slept the whole time."

She handed Rosy to me, and a surge of love rushed through my heart. I finally had my daughter in my arms, and I immediately knew that it was all worth it. We kissed her, inspected her, and cried.

My labor had been a five-and-a-half day nightmare. I had endured many things that I never could have imagined, and I laughed at the irony of them calling it a "natural birth." My mom said that if she had not been there, she never would have believed my birth story. But it was finally over.

We were able to check out of the hospital that evening, so that I could go home and recover. I soon realized that, although labor was done, the struggles were not over. Rosy was very happy to snuggle and sleep in my arms, but as I went to nurse her, she didn't respond. She just kept snuggling. I thought that she was also exhausted from the long ordeal. I held her and we both slept.

When we woke up, I tried again to feed her, but she just wanted to sleep. I got out her new little clothes and dressed her up, hoping that would stimulate her enough to realize she was hungry. It didn't work.

I struggled through the night, trying to nurse Rosy. I cried, and she cried. But she never latched on. I eventually realized that she did not have a rooting reflex or a latching reflex. I never imagined anything but blissful nursing. I lost out on all that I had thought my labor would be. Would I not be able to nurse my baby either?

By the next day, it was clear that we would have to intervene. She had been at my breast most of her short life, but since she hadn't latched on, we knew she hadn't gotten anything. We discussed our options with Irma, and she mentioned different formulas, goat's milk, and bottle styles.

After several days, we realized that Rosy was tongue-tied. There was a small clinic nearby that accepted walk-ins. The doctor clipped the tie effortlessly. We had high hopes that this would fix the problem. But it didn't. It didn't result in a single change from Rosy.

I, however, wasn't ready to give up just yet, so I had my own idea--a breast pump. Irma agreed that would be best, but was concerned that I couldn't extract enough milk to keep up with the demand. We decided to purchase an electric pump and give it a try.

I prayed that after we got milk in her, she would figure out how to nurse. I didn't want her to have nipple confusion, so I didn't want to start her off with a bottle. I had Nathan pick up some medicine droppers.

My milk started to come in and we quickly realized that I would have plenty of milk. I filled the dropper with milk and put it in Rosy's mouth. She responded right away. I was able to feed her enough to satisfy her and she fell into a contented sleep.

After Rosy woke, I eagerly tried to nurse her again. But she would have none of it. I pumped again and carefully fed her with the dropper. This was just the beginning of the cycle. Every three hours I pumped, attempted to nurse, fed her, washed the pump and prepared it for the next time. The whole routine took two hours. Then I slept for an hour and started the whole process again.

We continued this pattern for a full two weeks. Eventually, I was able to reduce the routine to one and a half hours, but it still needed to be done every three hours. I finally realized that she was not going to be nursing anytime soon, and I was ready to give the bottle a try.

Rosy spit out the bottle at first, but took to it pretty quickly. Bottle feeding was so much quicker than using the dropper. Since I started only attempting to nurse her a couple times a day, rather than around the clock, we were able to cut the time involvement down significantly. I was finally able to rest.

We headed back to our home up in the mountains. I stocked up on batteries so I could still use my breast pump on the days that there wasn't electricity. I went over to the bookshelf to find a book to read while pumping, and I saw it! It was the book about no pain in labor. I instantly felt the resentment surge up. I had been deceived. This book gave me false hope and set me up for a shocking disappointment. I picked up the book, looked at it, and threw it across the room.

Life settled down into a more manageable routine, but I wasn't willing to give up breastfeeding my baby. We still worked at it every single day! By six weeks, she was a chubby healthy baby, and she finally latched on for her first time ever.

Once Rosy latched on, I knew she could do it. I began the transition, and within a week, we had her fully transitioned from bottle to breast. I packed away my pump, bottles and other supplies, and sewed myself a nursing cape. Life was finally becoming what I had imagined--for a little while, at least!

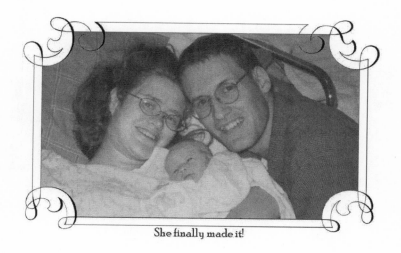

She finally made it!

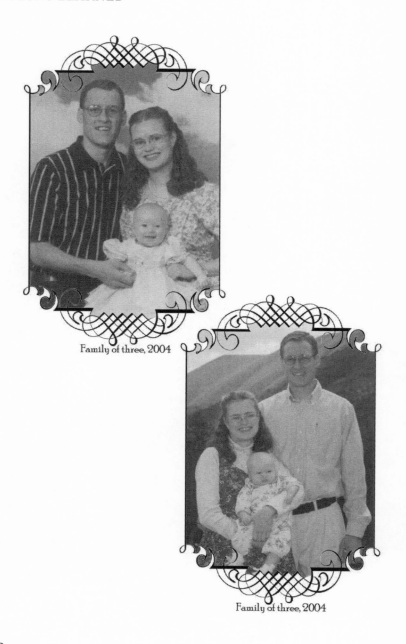

Family of three, 2004

Family of three, 2004

Chapter Four

Suddenly One Morning

I was loving my new life as a mother. Because I had so many younger siblings, I had plenty of experience taking care of a little one. So I found the daily chores of diapers, baths, changing clothes, etc. a breeze. I quickly got back into a new routine of daily life that included Rosy. Now that I had her, I didn't have nearly so much time to get bored. When I was first married, my to-do list would end by lunchtime and not pick up again until supper prep. Adding in a baby filled up my days nicely, but I still had enough time to work on sewing projects and letter writing.

One day when Rosy was just a few months old, I started feeling nauseous. We had enjoyed a potluck after church, and since we didn't have electricity at the church, I figured that something I had eaten must have gotten a little off while waiting to be served. That was a common occurrence, and I knew from experience I would be fine the next day. But I wasn't.

The nausea continued for several days. It started as a twinge in my stomach, but gradually became worse. Pretty soon, I was throwing up. "I hope you don't get this stomach bug," I told Nathan. "I hope I don't either," he replied. "I am way too busy to get sick!" And he didn't.

I, on the other hand, kept getting worse. I started to notice other symptoms, and I started having a nagging suspicion. But there was no way I could be pregnant, was there? Rosy was way too young.

I had bought a bulk package of twenty-five pregnancy tests when I was expecting Rosy, and I had a few left over. I tried to tell myself that I was crazy to even suspect that, but once the thought crossed my mind, there was no turning back. I dug out the tests from the back of a box and headed off to the bathroom.

Minutes later, I stared in surprise at two clearly defined lines. I was indeed pregnant! I quickly did the math. My babies would be thirteen months apart!

I had mixed emotions. On one side, I wanted to jump for joy for this new life, but the trials of so many losses and complications were so fresh. I was afraid of another loss, and I was afraid of not being able to be a good mother to Rosy if something went wrong.

It only took a split second for the joy to override any concern. I quickly decided to rejoice in the good news of today, and leave tomorrow's concerns for tomorrow.

I tried to imagine fun and exciting ways to announce a pregnancy to Nathan, but I am not naturally creative. I wasn't about to wait any longer than I needed to wait to tell. Nathan was just outside the bathroom, kneeling beside our bed, reading the Bible. I rushed out exclaiming, "I'm pregnant," as I shoved the stick in front of him.

Nathan's eyes widened in surprise. He ran his hand through his hair. "Well how about that," he said, and his face broke into a big grin. I threw myself into his arms and we laughed at the response we knew we would get.

The reality of the situation became very real very quickly, as the morning sickness did not restrict itself to just morning, nor did it stay within the first trimester. I was throwing up at least fifteen times a day again, and that was so much harder to deal with while taking care of a baby. My weight dropped off quickly. I don't know how much weight I lost, but I started the pregnancy at 115 pounds, and it was over four months before I saw that weight again.

I could barely eat. The only foods that sounded decent were the same few foods I had eaten when expecting Rosy--mostly junk.

One day, I noticed that Rosy was getting agitated when I would nurse her. It picked up with each feeding, and I knew something was wrong. I soon realized that she wasn't getting enough milk. I spent the next three days focusing on feeding her all day, in hopes of increasing my milk supply. Instead, my milk dried up and she wasn't wetting.

We agonized over what to do. I had worked so hard to develop a good nursing relationship with Rosy and since these two would be so close, I had assumed that I would tandem nurse. But my milk dried up abruptly and completely, so we had no recourse.

I didn't want to go with formula, so I researched and decided to feed her goat's milk. We added molasses to the milk for extra minerals and she loved it and thrived.

Finally the sickness settled and I was starting to show. We took a trip to Georgia for my brother's wedding. There was a stark difference between this trip and the last. When we last visited, I had suffered two losses and had no hope; this time I held one in my arms and carried another inside. I basked in the many congratulations, and praised God for His mercy and goodness to us.

We made it home and I anxiously awaited the sonogram that would reveal whether we were having a girl or a boy. The day arrived quickly and we headed down the bumpy road towards the city. I had mixed emotions. I wanted my daughter to have a brother, and I knew I wanted boys. Yet I also wanted her to have a sister close in age. I didn't get a sister until I was seventeen years old, and I wanted Rosy to experience what I had missed. I knew I would be happy either way though.

On the way for the sonogram we discussed names. We couldn't decide on boy names, but we agreed on a girl's name. "I guess it will just have to be a girl," Nathan joked. We held hands and laughed as we walked into the office together.

Dr. Quintana was ready for us so we didn't have to wait long. Just minutes later, she made her announcement, "It's another girl!" Nathan squeezed my hand and smiled. Everything looked great with the baby which was a relief.

We settled back into the car and I asked, "So, do we have a Susanna?"

"Actually," Nathan responded, "There is another name I have been thinking about that we should consider."

I was a little surprised, because I thought that "Susanna Ruth" was a done deal. But I was open to new ideas. "I'm thinking that I would like to name her Grace."

Hmm. I hadn't even thought of that name, but I knew I liked it. "Well, then, let's go with Grace." And that was that.

I loved to call my babies by name. For me, that is when the real bonding takes place. I love my babies before that, but once they have a name, they feel more like a specific individual.

Everything was looking perfect until I reached twenty-five weeks. I was working on my normal housework when I first felt it. I felt sick. "No, please no," I moaned, "it can't be!"

I brushed it off and kept going about my work. I felt it again, and I wanted to throw up. Surely this was only Braxton Hicks. Everybody had assured me that most people who had preterm labor only had it once.

I decided to lie down on my bed and write a letter. I didn't have any more contractions and I was relieved. But when I got up to prepare supper, I had another, and another, and yet another. The contractions picked up over the next couple of days and there was no doubt.

I was put back on bed rest, but this time I had more to think about than just me. I had a newly crawling baby. Our full-size bed was in a corner, so I lay on the edge and sat Rosy in the empty space between me and the wall. I made sure she had books and toys and she did beautifully.

Every day Nathan would make sure I had everything I needed on the table next to me. I used powdered goat's milk during the day, so I could mix it up from bed. He left food ready for me, and I would eat it cold in bed. Having a nine-month-old baby to entertain made bed rest much less boring, but it came with challenges as well.

We were very hesitant to go back on the medication that the doctor had given me for preterm labor with Rosy. We had discovered that it hadn't been used in the United States for twenty years, and that it was known for stalling labor in first-time moms. I just wasn't willing to risk that again, so we researched and learned that magnesium and calcium are muscle relaxants and help prevent contractions.

Without having a computer in our home, our research was limited, but we decided to give this a try. I stayed down on bed rest and took the supplements faithfully. It seemed to be working well. As long as I took the supplements and didn't move much, the contractions seemed under control.

After being on bed rest for a while, Nathan's sister, Deb, came to stay with us. It was perfect timing, because Rosy was reaching the point that she could no longer stay in one place on the bed all day long. She was thrilled for her freedom and I was grateful for hot meals again!

We went back in for a doctor's appointment and had another sonogram. The doctor said everything was going great. As long as things didn't get worse, she was comfortable with us continuing on as we were.

Four days later I woke with a start. "That was a strong contraction!" I thought. But then I had another, and another. I took more magnesium and calcium and drank a big glass of water. The contractions kept coming and were getting stronger. I started timing and, within an hour, at 5:00 a.m., I woke Nathan up.

"We need to go back in to the doctor," I told him. We had just been and he was a little hesitant--until he saw the contractions that I was having. These were different than the ones I had been battling. These were the real thing.

We packed our bags, expecting to stay in Arteaga for another month, so we would be closer to the doctor. We dropped off Deb and Rosy at the house and went on into town. Dr. Quintana checked me over and said that I was already at four centimeters and that it was too late to stop labor. She was going to be born today.

I cried, afraid for my baby. I knew she wasn't ready. I wasn't ready either. The due date we had written down put me at thirty-three weeks, but it was possible that we were up to two weeks off, since we didn't catch the pregnancy right off.

Dr. Quintana laid it out straight. She did not have the facilities to take care of a preemie. I could be admitted now, and they would take Gracie by ambulance to a larger hospital nearby, while I stayed there. Or, I could transfer now and birth at the bigger hospital.

LESSONS LEARNED

I felt safe in Dr. Quintana's small clinic. I had heard many stories and I was afraid of the bigger Mexican hospital. She said that she could still deliver me there, but she would not be my main caretaker. I knew that I couldn't have them take my baby somewhere else after birth, so we felt we had no choice.

The drive from the clinic to the hospital was fifteen minutes of torture. Cars were making their way to work, creating much traffic. We later found out that during that ride, I had gone from four centimeters to nine. No wonder that ride was so miserable!

We arrived at the hospital and they took me back right away. The nurse sent Nathan to the front to do paperwork, and she wanted me to go ahead and get prepped for birth. I asked if I could wait for Nathan, but she said I needed to go now.

We headed down the hall, and when we reached the doorway, she told me that my shoes weren't allowed past that point. I was wearing tennis shoes, tied in a double knot. I stared down at my feet. It had been at least a couple of months since I had taken those shoes off by myself, and she wanted me to do it alone, during transition, while standing??? I tried to get them off with my feet and then cried in frustration through the next contraction. There was no way I was getting all the way down there. Finally the nurse huffed and knelt down to remove my shoes. She handed them to me and led me to a small room.

The nurse handed me a gown and told me to change. I tried to get my shirt off, but another contraction hit and I stopped to breathe. "Take your shirt off NOW," the nurse snapped. The contraction had subsided, so I complied.

I lay on the bed the nurse indicated and asked her what she was doing. "I am going to give you an enema," she responded. I sat up abruptly and another contraction hit. "No, I don't need an enema," I managed to say. "You don't have an option," was her heartless reply.

Another nurse popped in and said that she wanted to check me before we finished. I was relieved, but surprised when she announced that I was already at nine centimeters. "Skip the enema, there is not enough time."

The first nurse huffed and told me to gather my stuff. She led me down the hall and we met Nathan coming back. I threw myself into his arms. "Promise me you won't leave me," I begged, and I started crying again.

Nathan held me as we headed down the hall. When we reached the double doors, the nurse turned to Nathan and announced, "No men are allowed past this point. You have to wait here."

They led me back to the labor room. Though surrounded by other laboring women, I felt so alone. I was scared to go through another birth, yet I was even more scared for the life of my baby. The uncertainty of not knowing if my baby was going to be OK made this so much harder to bear!

The doctors here had their list of duties and went on with their birth prep work without asking me anything or even explaining what they were going to do. I had never been in this type of medical setting before. I was used to being in control, and now I felt helpless.

Labor continued and they rushed me to the delivery room. Once again, I had a room full of people--both males and females. I didn't even bother to ask who they were this time. Dr. Quintana arrived, and I was so relieved. I finally had someone who cared about me there! This labor was so different from my first. It had been less than five hours since I first woke up. Labor went quickly and within a half hour Gracie was born.

They touched her head to my lips and, before I could even respond, they whisked her away. I did not know that it would be two weeks before I would even hold her.

Dr. Quintana focused on me, while some of the others left to take care of Gracie. I still needed to deliver the placenta and be stitched up from the episiotomy. I asked about Gracie and she knew nothing other than that she was alive and "looked good." She only had a brief glance, herself, so she couldn't say much.

One of the nurses came back to tell me that Gracie was 1800 kilograms or 3 lb., 9 ounces and was breathing on her own. How tiny! But I was relieved to know she was breathing. And I had gone from a five-day labor with Rosy to a five-hour labor with Grace.

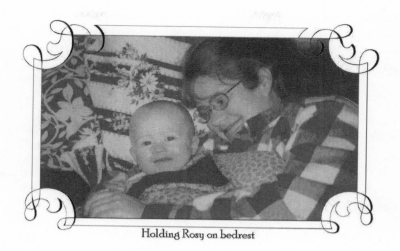

Holding Rosy on bedrest

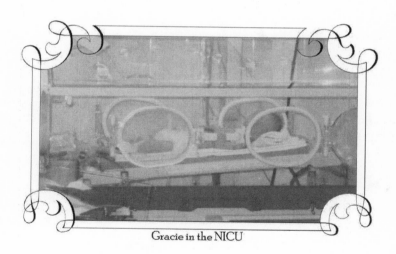

Gracie in the NICU

Chapter Five

God Giveth More Grace

Dr. Quintana finished her work and had to go. She apologized for leaving me while I was still in the delivery room, but she had to go back to her birth center. I was left alone. I started shaking.

A man came and wheeled me out and left me in an empty hallway. I was freezing and the trembling was increasing. I'd had nothing to eat or drink since I woke up, and so much had happened since then. I was left on that little cot without anything to cover me, and it was an hour before I saw anyone. Finally, a nurse walked by and I asked for a blanket and water. She handed me a small disposable cup, filled halfway with lukewarm water and left.

When the nurse returned, I asked again for a blanket and more water. This time she gave me a sheet, but no water. "Where is my husband?" I asked. "I need my husband!" She grunted and walked away. I continued trembling violently.

I found out later that Nathan was just on the other side of the door, pacing and waiting for me to be brought out. I was left in that hallway for several hours. It felt like the loneliest time of my life.

I could smell food cooking. I was starving and it smelled so good. I couldn't wait to eat. I could tell they had made a hot meal. Finally an attendant came to take me to a room. He explained that there had been a delay in getting a room for me because they had to clean it from the last patient. I asked about Nathan and he was surprised that no one had taken me to him.

He walked me through the doorway, and there he was! I held my hands up and Nathan hugged me. I asked about Gracie, but Nathan didn't know any more than I did. We passed several carts of lunch plates and it looked as good as it smelled!

Once I got to my room and settled down, I was really starving! I waited for lunch to be brought, but it never came. I asked about it, and the attendant said he would ask. When a nurse came in, I asked her about lunch. Everybody told me they would ask about it. I kept waiting. I found out later that I didn't arrive to my room until it was too late to be placed on the lunch list, so they skipped me.

The nurse came to do an IV and she botched it. My hand turned green and purple. She insisted on continuing to try in the same spot because it was easier for her to have it on that side.

Dr. Quintana came back later to fill us in on the hospital rules. Gracie would be in the room with all the other preemies, and they did not allow any parents to go in. They kept the curtains closed most of the time, but we were allowed to stand up and look at her through the window for an hour twice a day. That was also the only time we would be able to speak to her doctor and ask any questions.

We also needed to purchase any supplies she would need. Each evening the nurse would give us a list of what she would need the next day, and we would purchase the feeding tubes, IVs, and all the other items that it seemed like a hospital would provide.

That evening, they wheeled me up to look at her for the first time. I could look through the big window into a small nurses' station and through another window past that. Gracie was another twenty feet beyond that, in an incubator. I wanted to pick her up and hold her, kiss her, and tell her that I loved her. But I couldn't.

Gracie was so tiny. She was long for her size and extremely thin. Her skin draped over her face, and her long arms and legs looked disproportionate. I asked about nursing her, and they told me that she was too small and would not be able to nurse yet. They would be feeding her with a tube, and if I could pump, they would use my milk.

I got up to take a shower. After helping me to the bathroom, Nathan went back to visit with my mother, who had arrived a few minutes earlier. The nurse came in the room and demanded to know where I was. Nathan told her that I was in the shower and she was hopping mad. I listened to her from behind the closed door, afraid she was going to come in and get me back into bed. My mom kept her talking while Nathan came back to help me get ready to go back out. The nurse shot daggers at me while she chewed me out.

Finally, suppertime came around. I had been up since 4:00 a.m., given birth, and still hadn't had any food. Lunch had looked so good, but when supper arrived, I was sorely disappointed. The dry crusty white bread had been slathered in mayo (my most despised food ever), with a thin piece of sandwich meat and a piece of processed cheese. It was the most pitiful looking sandwich I had ever seen. Next to it was a Jell-o cup. This was so far from the meal I had seen at lunch. It was hard to be grateful for this food--it was such a letdown. The only redeeming factor was the apple and cup of milky oatmeal.

I was so relieved to sleep that night!

"Knock, knock." I woke with a start. One of the doctors came into our room to tell us that Gracie was struggling to breathe on her own. She needed surfactant to help keep her lungs from collapsing. Normally, they would not administer the medications until we went to the pharmacy to purchase it, but the pharmacy was closed and time was of the essence.

The doctor offered to use the dose he had on hand, if we promised that we would purchase another and replace it first thing in the morning. We quickly agreed. He reminded us that we would not be able to take Gracie home until the bill was paid in full, and if we didn't replace this, it would be added to the tab.

The next morning, they released me in time to go up and see Gracie. The surfactant had done its job and she was breathing again. That midnight dose had likely saved her life.

We headed back to the house in Arteaga where Nathan's sister and Rosy were waiting. I hugged my bigger baby as I cried for my little baby. We loaded up our belongings in the car and headed to our friends' house. They lived very close to the hospital, so we would be staying there while we were going back and forth to the hospital.

That night I sobbed for hours. My heart was breaking. I never imagine having to leave my new little baby alone. I finally fell into a fitful sleep, but I didn't get much rest at all.

By the time we arrived at the hospital the next morning, I had only been able to pump a few drops, as my milk hadn't let down yet. I knew that the colostrum came in tiny amounts, but I had pumped and pumped. While looking at those drops, I felt like a complete failure.

Gracie was on the third floor, and I knew that there was no way I was going up any stairs. We headed up the elevator ramps. The ramps went back and forth and they could be too steep. To a newly postpartum woman, those ramps felt as though they stretched on for miles. One of my big memories through Gracie's hospital stay was walking, walking, walking and feeling like I would never make it.

The next two weeks are still a blur in my mind. We went back and forth to the hospital, and I pumped, pumped, pumped. Within a few days, I was pumping enough for

Gracie to have all she needed and to start making bottles for Rosy, too. I was happy to be able to provide that nourishment to Rosy again, even if it was via bottle.

Gracie needed oxygen at first, and then bilirubin lights. Quickly, she was stable in every way. Now she just needed to grow. We had a sonogram picture of Gracie sucking her thumb. I watched through the window as she would try to suck her thumb again. She kept whacking herself in the head with the board attached to her arm, there to prevent her from pulling out her IV. She cried, and so did I.

Eleven days after Gracie was born we had a mini party. Rosy was turning one! Yes, my two little girls were Irish twins! Rosy was too little to understand what was going on, and she was not allowed in the hospital.

By now, the doctor told us that there were two things that Gracie needed to do in order to be able to go home: nurse well and gain weight. During the first couple of days, Gracie had lost down to an even three pounds, and now she was slowly climbing. Every day they told us how many grams she had gained.

I was anxious to begin nursing her, but the hospital insisted that they needed to monitor her food intake. Gracie was fed with a feeding tube for the first week, and then they switched her to a bottle to see if she would be able to take it. She sucked fine, but she would tire before she finished her milk. The next few days, they fed her the bottle and then topped it off with the feeding tube.

All preemie care was done during non-visiting hours. While we were there, the nurses would tell me about how great she was doing or share some of her antics. While I was grateful that they were gracious enough to share those details, I struggled with jealousy. I should be the one holding my baby. I should be the one caring for her.

Every day, I asked if I could nurse her. Day after day, they said she wasn't ready. We were at the hospital from 10:00-11:00 am and from 4:00-5:00 pm every day. Finally, on the thirteenth day, the doctor said Gracie was ready to try to nurse. She told me to be there at 6:00 a.m. for her morning feeding.

I was jumping for joy inside. I would FINALLY be able to hold my baby. The next morning, they placed little Gracie in my arms. I held her, kissed her, stroked her face, and told her that her mommy loved her. She snuggled right up.

"Hurry up and feed her." The nurse startled me. "You can't let her sleep yet, we need to keep her on schedule."

I lifted her up to nurse, and she latched on instantly. What joy to finally nurse my baby! She nursed like a pro. All the nurses and doctors had to see, and they would all randomly lift up the blanket to check and see if she was still latched on correctly.

It was a very awkward situation, as I was very modest by nature. But I knew that if I protested, I would lose the chance to nurse altogether. I decided not to let the embarrassment cloud my joy of feeding my baby.

After she nursed, Gracie pulled back and fell into a contented sleep. I tried to keep her in the same position and not let on that she was done. I wanted every minute I could with my little one. They quickly figured out that she was done and took her away.

After the doctors left, the nurse asked if I would like to change Gracie's diaper. I relished every moment!

I was reluctant to hand my daughter over. Once I got her, I didn't want to give her up. The nurse told me that I needed to be there at 6:00 a.m., 9:00 a.m., 12:00 p.m., 6:00 p.m. and 9:00 p.m., to feed her. We also needed to be there from 10:00-11:00 a.m. and 4:00-5:00 p.m. for the visiting time.

We thought that we would replace the two hours standing in front of the window with the feeding time, but they said we needed to stay the entire visiting hours. In the morning hour, the doctor gave us an overview of how things were going. In the evening, he gave us a list of the supplies we needed for the next day. The doctors were not able to change their schedule to provide that information during the feeding hours.

The next few days were crazy. Sometimes Nathan left me at the hospital from one feeding to the next, but we didn't like that option. There was nowhere for me to wait but on the floor of a hallway. I carried some books with me, but I hated sitting alone at the hospital with nothing to do. I would rather be back at our friends' house with Rosy.

After a couple of days, it felt like this schedule would kill us. Gracie was nursing great and she was stable. The only thing keeping her there was her weight--or lack thereof.

We prayed about our options and talked to the doctor. We felt like Gracie really needed her mother's care to thrive, and Rosy really needed her family back together. We asked the doctor about bringing her home now.

First, the doctor reminded us that they could not give her to us until we had paid her bill and mine in full. Gracie was still tiny, but the doctor was so impressed with how she was doing. "I cannot recommend that you take her home this small," the doctor told us "But I will give my permission and I believe that she will do just fine."

That was the confirmation that we needed! Nathan started gathering the money we needed. He took the money we had on us and emptied the bank account. My mom had given us some money, and a few days later, my dad had given us some more. We added it all together, but it still wasn't enough.

We wanted to take Gracie home the next morning, and now, the only thing holding us back was finances. "God, if it is your will for us to bring Gracie home now," we prayed, "please provide the rest of the money."

I went to bed feeling sick at the thought of money keeping my baby away from me, but Nathan held me and reminded me to trust. The next morning, we were getting ready to head to the hospital when a friend came and handed us an envelope. He said his church wanted to help with Gracie's expenses.

Once we were in the car, I ripped into the envelope and counted the handful of bills. God had provided just what we needed to bring Gracie home!

When we got to the hospital, instead of going to feed Gracie right away, we stopped at the office. The secretary handed us a "Paid in full" receipt and congratulated us! That little slip of paper felt more valuable than gold-- it was the ticket to bring home our daughter.

The nurses gathered up all of Gracie's things and said their goodbyes, while the doctor gave us last minute instructions. Gracie was placed in my arms, and this time I wouldn't have to say goodbye. My heart felt full!

We headed out with our little daughter weighing 3 lb. 15 oz. We spent the next couple of months at the house in Arteaga, as our home in the mountain was just too cold and ventilated for such a wee little one.

I kept Gracie against my chest and wrapped her up in my jacket. She practically lived in my jacket until she was about eight weeks old and about six pounds.

Every other day, we walked across the street to the little tiendita, a Mexican corner store. We draped a clean blanket over the produce scale and checked her weight. Everyone cheered her on as we watched her weight gradually increase.

It only took Gracie a few days to get into a nursing schedule that worked for her. She was still not able to nurse enough to keep her tiny tummy full an entire three hours, so she nursed every two hours around the clock. I was exhausted, but I was content.

Rosy was thrilled with her new baby sister. She loved to cuddle up with us, and she was sure that I had brought her a little baby doll of her own.

The first few months, Gracie just ate and slept, cuddled and cooed. Eventually, I realized that something was wrong. At first everyone thought I was crazy to even suspect, but my mother's instinct told me that I couldn't let it go. When Gracie was four months old, she was confirmed to be completely blind. Thus began the doctor appointments and all that went along with that, but that is another story.

I really struggled physically after Gracie was born. Five pregnancies, two births, and months of bed rest in such quick succession left my body weary and worn. It took me a year to recover.

When the dishes needed to be washed, I filled the sink with hot soapy water, gathered all the dishes, scraped the leftovers into the trash, and added the dishes to my water. Then I was exhausted so I would let the dishes soak while I rested.

When I cooked supper, I would need to lie down and rest before I felt the strength to sit up at the table to eat. Life with two children so young was much harder than I expected. I thought I would be the energetic mom, who could do it all, but in reality, I could barely care for my children, and I couldn't keep up with my house. What would life hold next?

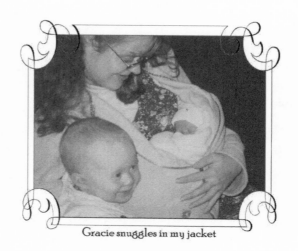

Gracie snuggles in my jacket

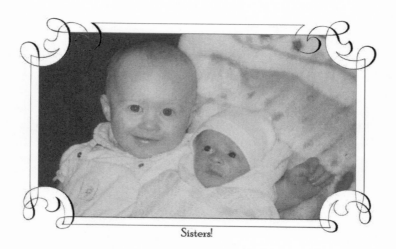

Sisters!

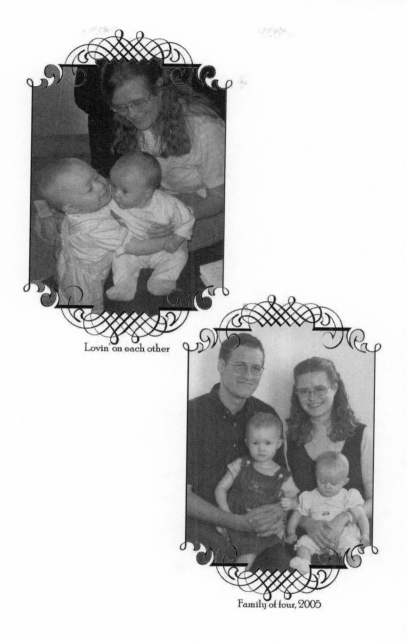

Lovin' on each other

Family of four, 2005

Chapter Six

Man Plans His Way

Life took on a whole new change as God led us to leave Mexico and return to Nathan's home town. We left when Gracie was fourteen months and Rosy had just turned two.

As we were packing up our house, I realized that I felt worse than normal. I thought that I was exhausted from the extra work load, but when I lay on the concrete floor after our bed had been loaded, I knew it was much more. Nathan took me to my parents' house. I was trembling violently and my fever shot up. I could tell that the girls were starting to feel off as well. That first day, I was too weak to even hold them. I was glad my mom was there!

Nathan packed up all of our belongings into a six-foot trailer, and we decided to head on out--sick or not. We planned to make our cross country trip in just a couple of days, but shortly after we left, Nathan came down with the dreaded illness, too.

It took us four days, but we finally made it to Flagler, Colorado. By that point Nathan and I were starting to mend, but we knew the girls needed help. Nathan's family came over to help us unload and we took the girls to the doctor. They were admitted to the hospital and diagnosed with influenza. What a way to start our new life in the United States.

During Gracie's sickness and hospital stay, she nursed very little. Although she was fourteen months old, because of her other challenges, Gracie was still totally breastfed. She could not tolerate any solids whatsoever. My milk supply was dwindling, and we considered our options. I knew that I would need to pull out the pump to get it back up. Instead, we decided that it was time to wean so that I could work towards healing my body without concern for how it could affect Gracie.

We switched Gracie from the breast to a bottle with very little effort. While she was sick and too weak to nurse, she was able to suck on the bottle. She saw it as a relief, rather than a poor substitute. I think the switch was harder for me than for her.

We felt like my body really needed some time to heal. For the first time, we questioned some of the things that we believed about having children. We knew that children were a blessing from the Lord, but was there ever a justifiable reason to prevent them?

We struggled with that question, and concern for my physical situation won over any arguments. We decided to use a barrier method to prevent pregnancy for a while to give my body some time to get stronger. I was hoping for a full year of recovery without being pregnant or nursing.

Nine months went by and we felt like we were in control of the decision to postpone children, but God, in His sovereignty, chose to override our plans. I am reminded of Proverbs 16:9, "A man's heart plans his way, But the LORD directs his steps." We thought we knew the way we should go, but God had better plans for us!

When I first suspected that I was pregnant, I fretted. I didn't think I should be, but my body was telling me differently. I called Nathan, asking him to bring home a test. He didn't think I could be pregnant either, but he brought the test home, just to appease me.

I took the test and it appeared negative. I breathed a sigh of relief, yet also felt a twinge of disappointment. I went to bed with mixed emotions.

In the early hours of the morning, I stepped into the bathroom. As I walked through the door, I stopped short. "What!" I gasped, and ran over to see the test on the counter. There they were; two lines.

Because the test didn't show up in the time frame, I felt I needed another to confirm it. I paced around all day wondering whether I was really pregnant or not. I took another test the next morning, and this one left no doubt. I was indeed pregnant!

We had tried to prevent, but God had had the last word! It only took a split second for my doubts to turn to joy! We were excited about a new little one.

LESSONS LEARNED

Shortly after I found out we were pregnant, we planned to move again, though I thoroughly enjoyed my life in small-town Flagler. Nathan wanted to start a Bible Study with the Hispanics in the area, but they mostly lived in a town about forty-five miles away.

We rented a mobile home in Limon, Colorado, and Nathan applied for a job at the meat processing plant where most of the Hispanics worked. We felt that he could have a greater level of influence if he worked alongside them.

Morning sickness was so much better this time around. I was still throwing up and felt yucky, but this time it was a much more tolerable level. We packed up our house and headed to Limon.

I found a midwife in Colorado Springs and was hopeful that I could finally have my homebirth. I thought that maybe since my body had had a larger break, it would be strong enough to carry the baby full term. But at the same time, I felt leery.

I loved having real midwife visits, and I loved how they looked at the whole picture of my pregnancy and health, rather than just the small window of the medical perspective.

Soon it was time for the big sonogram! We drove to the city and stopped at Walmart on our way. "This is the cutest outfit I have ever seen!" I explained to Nathan, holding up a newborn suit. "Look at the little vest and bow tie! Can we get it? Please?" I begged.

Nathan laughed and reminded me that we didn't even know if it was a boy or girl. "Just in case," I pleaded.
80

"Please!" Up till now, I had never purchased a new outfit for either of my girls. They had only worn gifts or hand-me-downs. But something about this little man suit drew me in!

"I'll tell you what," Nathan conceded, "If the sonogram shows we are having a boy, we will come back and get it."

I threw my arms around Nathan's neck and kissed him. "And I'll hold you to it," I pronounced with a twinkle in my eye.

We never made it back to Walmart, but I wasn't disappointed. As much as I thought it would be great to have a boy, it only took a split second to be excited about the prospect of three girls!

Once again I went back to the name we had previously chosen--Susanna Ruth--but Nathan wasn't interested this time. We discussed names the whole way home, and settled on Elizabeth Anne. Elizabeth was quickly dubbed Lizzie.

We both wanted a Bible name for her first name, and we chose Anne in honor of my dad. He always told me that he wanted a granddaughter named "Anne with an E," and we knew that the "E" was an essential part of her name!

I was only nineteen weeks when I first felt the contractions. "Oh, God, please let this just be Braxton Hicks," I prayed. I did not include, "Not my will but thine be done." I wanted my will to be His will.

I'd learned before that God's ways are not always my ways, and we were facing that again. The contractions continued to pick up. They were just enough to make us really concerned, but not enough to be positive that this was true preterm labor.

My midwife recommended some herbal tinctures and told me to make sure I drank plenty of water. That helped for a while, but eventually, I was not able to keep the contractions under control. Finally, my midwife told me that I needed to be under a doctor's care. However, if I could make it to thirty-six weeks, she would still deliver my baby.

I began calling doctors, but no one would take me. Most doctors had a deadline for taking pregnant patients, and I was just passed that point. I felt scared and hopeless.

"Nathan, I'm afraid that I will end up losing Lizzie all together if I have a preemie birth and no one to care for us." Nathan assured me that we would find someone. Finally, my midwife was able to get me in with a doctor who made an exception to the cut-off.

By this point, it was clear that this was indeed preterm labor. After Gracie's preemie birth, I wasn't willing to take any chances. I was going to do anything they recommended.

They prescribed Terbutaline and recommended bed rest. My dad knew a young lady, Michelle, whom he thought might be able to come help me for a while. He contacted Michelle, and after a few emails back and forth, she agreed to come to stay with me the remainder of the pregnancy.

Nathan took me to his parents' house, so I could stay there during the day, while we waited for Michelle to get there. We got the Terbutaline and I took my first dose. Pretty soon, everything got fuzzy, I felt hot and dizzy, and it got harder and harder to breathe. I was trembling. I could hear my mother-in-law in the background, trying to talk to me, but I zoned her out.

I put my hand on my heart and I could feel it pounding. Everything around me started spinning. My body felt flush, and my limbs went limp. "Breathe, Misty, Breathe," I told myself. But it was so hard. I closed my eyes, leaned back, and put all my energy into trying to get air.

Eventually my chest loosened up and my breathing was less labored. My head started to clear, and I could hear my mother-in-law saying something about calling 911. That brought me to, quickly, and I finally responded to her.

"I'm OK," I got out, "wait." And I closed my eyes again. I just focused on breathing for a little longer, as the feeling began to dissipate.

Soon, most of the trouble passed, and I was just a little weak and shaky. My mother-in-law called the doctor for me. He said that this was a side effect of the medicine and I would be fine. My mother-in-law explained how badly I had responded and they agreed to change it up a little. They prescribed a slow release version of the pill, so my body wasn't given such a rush of it at once.

The slow release pill was only once a day, but it also slowly released the symptoms, and for the remainder of the pregnancy, I would have smaller repeats of this same incident every day.

Michelle arrived and took over all the tasks that were falling apart. We hit it off quickly, and it was the beginning of a long-term friendship. I was so glad to have someone to stay on top of the girls! They were only two and three and they needed much more care than I could give them.

I was at twenty-eight weeks when my contractions started increasing even more. Nathan and I fretted about whether I should go into the hospital or not. It was a two-hour trip, so we only wanted to go if it were necessary. We finally decided to go.

They performed a fetal fibronectin test, which would tell us if birth was imminent. The test was negative, so there was a good chance that we could stop the labor. A sonogram showed that I hadn't started dilating, so they increased my medication and sent me home.

The increased medication did slow things down, but not without a price tag. I also had increased side effects. I constantly felt like I was in a fog, and I would have flair-ups several times a day.

The doctor also asked that I get regular sonograms to measure the length of my cervix, so that we could be on top of things and know right away if there were any changes. I went from bed rest to getting out of the house twice a week. Michelle would get the kids all ready and drive me to the local hospital. I hated the transvaginal sonograms, but I was willing to do anything to prevent another preemie birth.

After each visit to the doctor, we waited anxiously to see if we would receive the call that there was a problem. By the time we were sure that they weren't calling, it was time to go in again. The technician was not allowed to tell me anything about the current results, but she always filled me in about the results of the previous.

Each sonogram showed slight change. My cervix was funneling, or dilating from the top, while still closed at the bottom.

Finally the day came when we got the call. "There have been more changes in your cervix, and we think that you should consider being admitted to the hospital." They also told me that if I went, I would not be going home until after birth.

This was hard to hear! I was only at thirty weeks. There were only two possible outcomes, and neither was good. I would either have a preemie or I would have an extended hospital stay. There was so much to consider!

I would be in Colorado Springs, and Michelle would have to take the girls to Flagler to stay with Nathan's parents. They would be 120 miles away, and I knew that I would not see them much. Nathan would be working in between the two. Each evening he would have to choose whether to go to the hospital and see me, or go to his parents' house and see Rosy and Gracie.

We prayed that God would make it clear, and He did. My contractions picked back up, and we knew that we couldn't prevent this birth on our own. I instructed from the couch while Nathan packed my bag, and Michelle packed for the girls.

I squeezed my girls tight, not wanting to let them go. Nathan led me to the car, while Michelle took the girls in the opposite direction. It felt like my family was splitting in two and my heart was breaking.

The hospital admitted me quickly and did another sonogram. My cervix was now paper thin and they said it was possible for the baby to be born any time. The nurse prepped me for a steroid shot, to help Lizzie's lungs develop. I cringed at the thought of another needle, but this was just the first of many. The goal was to keep Lizzie in, but we had to be ready for either outcome.

I was grateful that I did have access to the internet and was able to communicate with family and friends. I treasure those letters because they tell the story that is now mostly a blur in my mind. The drugs were so extensive that I can't remember most of the details, but thanks to good communication those details were not lost.

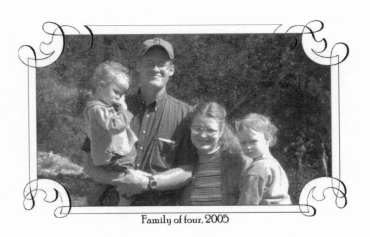

Family of four, 2005

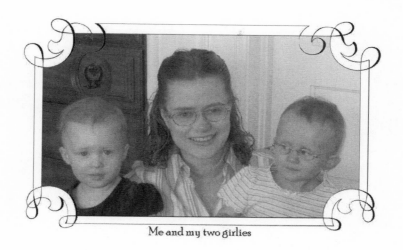

Me and my two girlies

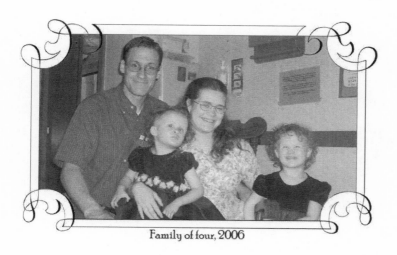

Family of four, 2006

87

Chapter Seven

Letters from the Hospital

April 17, 2007

Dear Momma,

I am having less contractions and premature labor symptoms here. Everything is so monitored and nipped in the bud. And when I need to sit up, I just press a button and the bed sits me up. There is nobody to knock or jolt me. Everything I need is within reach, so less leaning over. No more going to doctor appointments. All these things combined will help me to keep Elizabeth in longer than I could have at home.

If I had not come when I did, Elizabeth would probably be here now. ... We did another cervical length exam. On Thursday, they were very concerned that there was only one centimeter left closed. Now that centimeter is pretty much gone. We believe that happened on Friday, and birth could happen any time now. At this point, they will do whatever they can to try to stop labor. Please pray for me, as that won't be any fun.

They did the fetal fibronectin test when I first got here. They did it the last time I was here and it was negative. That meant that I probably wouldn't go into labor in the next two weeks. This time it was positive. That doesn't mean that I absolutely will give birth soon, but it greatly increases the probability, especially when you add in all of my other high risk factors. Fibronectin is some kind of protein in your uterus, and it won't show up until your body is getting ready to give birth.

I was worried about how the food would be here. It is very good. They don't just serve three meals. They give me a menu of everything they have, and it is quite a variety. I just call in room service and I can get whatever I want, whenever I want it, between 6:30 a.m. and 6:30 p.m. There are no limits or regulations about how much and how often. It is kind of nice. They have some good snacks, too-- lots of fruits and even plain yogurt. I could have steak and shrimp every day, if I wanted to. It's like a fancy hotel.

Right now I am hooked up to a bunch of monitors. They want to track contractions and Elizabeth's heartbeat for an hour. She is wiggling all around and keeps getting out from under the monitor.

Nathan spent the first night here with me. He left halfway through the day to go be with the girls. He won't be able to be here much, because the girls need him with them. I would love him to be here more, of course, but the girls need one of us with them as much as possible. It was very hard when he left, knowing that I wouldn't see him for days. We both cried a lot. But we will make it.

Please keep baby Elizabeth in your prayers. I am 31 ½ weeks now.

Also, Gracie is having a hard time without her Mommy. Now she is sick and threw up all night. I wish I could be with her. ... It was very hard to say goodbye to Nathan when he left the hospital.

Well, I'd better get my breakfast ordered. I'll write again when I have more news.

Love,

Misty

April 20, 2007

Hi Momma,

I had a rough evening again yesterday, but things are settled down now. I just hope they stay that way, because this is getting old.

I am supposed to be hooked to monitors every eight hours, and from start to finish, it takes close to an hour and a half each time. The nurses tend to stretch out the time in the morning and then take it from the night. So, I am getting four to five hours of sleep at night. Today is my sixth day here and I just can't take it anymore. If I don't get more sleep, I am going to fall apart.

Love,

Misty

April 22, 2007

Dear Grandma,

Friday, we had a surprisingly good day, with few contractions. However, yesterday made up for that. More contractions, more drugs. I also had a lot of lower back pain and cervical pressure and lost some of my mucous plug--all bad signs.

We are making it. Generally, I am getting through this ok. Yesterday, my family was here, which was great until they had to leave. Gracie was crying, and Rosy wouldn't give me a kiss. ... It just breaks my heart when they have to leave.

They will be coming again this afternoon, along with Nathan's family. But after that, they won't be able to come again until at least Thursday. That seems so long away. (Well, Nathan will come if Elizabeth comes.)

I just talked to my doctor. He's afraid that if we continue as we have been, Elizabeth will be born very soon. I have been taking one med (Procardia) on a regular basis, and Terbutaline as needed. While I have sort of adjusted to the Procardia, the Terbutaline really messes me up. The side effects are so miserable. Up till now, I have never had more than one a day, and have even skipped some days. Now ... I am going to have to start taking it four times a day, in addition to the Procardia. I don't know how I am going to handle this.

Please keep me in your prayers. I am feeling very discouraged right now. I DON'T want to take this junk. I talked to my doctor about the possibility of the effects of the drugs on her being worse than being born now. He said that if she is born now, she will get much more drugs in the NICU than she will be getting from the meds that I am taking, and that they would also have higher risks of potential side effects. What can I say? For Elizabeth's sake, I really don't have any option but to take them.

Love,

Misty

April 27, 2007

Dear Family and Friends,

Yesterday I woke up and knew I was in labor. It came fast and hard. I was sure that Elizabeth would be born any minute. Once again, they were able to stop it, and things settled down and the rest of the day went better.

I just found out that one of my medications will be tripled. They are doubling the amount per pill and I will be taking it six times a day, instead of four. My doctor wants to prevent labor from starting at this point, rather than keep stopping it. I am definitely not looking forward to seeing what the side effects of this will be.

Misty

May 5, 2007

Dear Family and Friends,

We did it! On Thursday we reached 34 weeks. Once that was a goal that we thought was impossible. Now we have passed. I am so grateful that God has given Elizabeth that extra time in my womb.

Since they increased my medication, the threats of Elizabeth being born have greatly reduced. Yesterday I did have a few more contractions than I had had in the few days prior, but not enough to bring Elizabeth. Other premature labor symptoms have also reduced. Our new goal is 36 weeks.

Medication side effects are my biggest problem these days. Thinking is too hard now for me to write much. I am on day 22 at the hospital, and feel like I have moved in! I will be glad when we are able to go home!

Today, Nathan and the girls will come to spend the day with me. It will be great to see them!

Misty

May 7, 2007

Dear Family and Friends,

Greetings. After several relatively calm days, Elizabeth decided to give us some more excitement! I woke up this morning at 3:15 in hard labor. Contractions were coming 2

½ to 3 minutes apart. I was sure that we wouldn't be able to stop it this time. But, once again, I was wrong! Of course it did mean a pretty rough day with additional side effects from the extra drugs. But I am glad that we were able to buy Elizabeth some more time.

Now we would appreciate your prayers that God would give us wisdom. As we get farther along, we need to decide at what point we stop intervening if labor starts while still on the medication. And also at what point we stop all medications.

Today I had a Fetal Anatomy Sonogram. Elizabeth looks great. We haven't found any problems whatsoever. Her weight is estimated at 4 lb. 6 oz. (in comparison Gracie weighed 3 lb. 9 oz.). We are very pleased that she is growing so well.

I am 34 weeks, 5 days now. That really is a miracle, as at one point we didn't think that I would be able reach 30 weeks.

Sincerely,

Misty

May 13, 2007

Dear Momma,

Hey, Happy Mother's Day!!!!

LESSONS LEARNED

I almost had a Mother's Day baby. Last night, Elizabeth decided that she wanted to come. The nurses weren't sure if they were supposed to stop labor at this point. They got a labor and delivery nurse who checked me out and said that she would be born tonight (which was last night). Then they got in touch with the doctor who said to stop labor. So they did. I am feeling pretty yucky now. This morning Nathan said that we are not going to stop labor anymore. I will keep taking my daily medications until Wednesday night, but no more additional drugs. I almost wanted to do that last night. I was ready to get this over with!!! After what they gave me last night, I probably won't start labor again for several days anyway.

So today has been pretty rough, with not only the extra contractions all day long, but also the side effects from the drugs last night are still pretty bad. Sometimes I feel like I just can't handle any more. Please pray that God will give me the grace to make it through these next few days. Also, please pray that I will be able to get the rest I need. I might be in bed all day, but I'm having a hard time getting enough sleep. Part of it is that I am given medication several times a night, and I also miss my family most at night.

Well, I wanted to write more, but my head is pounding and the letters on the screen are blurring up.

I love you and can't wait to see you soon.

Love,

Misty

May 17, 2007

Dear Family and Friends,

Today we reached a milestone that we never imagined reaching–36 weeks! God has been good and given us more than we hoped for. At this point, it is very probable that Elizabeth would not need to stay in the NICU, but would come home when I do. This morning, I took my last pill. Once all the drugs are out of my system, we are expecting a quick birth.

I talked to my doctor this morning and asked him what was the soonest he had someone have their baby after stopping these medications, and he said 2-3 days. I was surprised, as I expected it to be much sooner than that. I should have asked that sooner, as to not set myself up for disappointment.

So, we are praying for a Thursday night or Friday birth, and that Elizabeth and I can go home on Saturday. I know that we cannot plan the timing, but I can hope and pray. Because of my situation, everybody at the hospital assumes that birth will be very soon.

Please pray that Elizabeth will have no health complications. They are not foreseeing any problems, but some things simply cannot be determined until birth. Elizabeth has been referred to as a picture perfect baby. She is extremely active and she has a reputation for kicking the monitors every time they try to listen to her heartbeat. When she gets tired of kicking it, she moves out from under it.

Please pray that today I can get some extra sleep. I have slept very little the last few days and am feeling exhausted

97

and that God will give me grace to accept His timing for Elizabeth's birth. Also, please pray that once I go into labor, Nathan will be able to make it to the hospital in time. And of course, I would appreciate your prayers for me during the labor and delivery!

I am so grateful for the many prayers that have been lifted up in my behalf and Elizabeth's as well. God has been good to surround me with so many people who love and care about us.

Sincerely,

Misty

May 19, 2007

I spent the day trying to get a nap, but my plan kept getting interrupted. I can't tell you how many times I was woken up after 3-5 minutes of sleep. But, I was able to get my monitoring done early, and I got to sleep about 9:30.

I had very few contractions yesterday, but they were pretty good between midnight and 1:30. Then they died off. So, I am going to try to get a nap this morning, and Michelle is bringing the girls this afternoon. They will all go back to Flagler this evening, including Nathan. He hasn't seen the girls since Wednesday evening, so they really need some Daddy time. And I haven't seen them since last Sunday. They will all come on Sunday after church, and Nathan will spend the night here again. Of course, plans will change if Elizabeth does come between now and then!

May 21, 2007

I've been telling Nathan that I felt like my stomach has really grown a lot this week. They weigh us once a week, and would you believe that I gained 4 lb.? I weigh 14 lb. more than the day before Rosy was born, and 24 lb. more than when Gracie was born. It will be interesting to see how long it takes to get the extra off. I am getting a double chin, and I can't give all the blame for that on pregnancy.

Misty

May 24, 2007

Dear Family and Friends,

Well, it looks like thing are starting to pick up. I had contractions on and off all night last night, and since early this morning they have been quite regular, varying from 2-8 minutes apart the whole day. They are not quite strong enough to say I am in labor, but there has definitely been progress. I don't know if it will continue like this for awhile, or if I will have Elizabeth in my arms by morning. Either one is a possibility.

I am excited about the possibility of the end being so close. I will be 37 weeks tomorrow. That is considered full term, so we have no concern for Elizabeth's health. I never would have imagined we would even get close to this point. I am so grateful that God gave Elizabeth the time that she needed in my womb. And now I am grateful that our family will be back together very soon.

99

LESSONS LEARNED

I have been able to get up little by little this past week. I am seeing improvement in my strength, but I am also seeing that recovery after nearly four months in bed will be very slow and long. I feel pretty good if I don't do anything, but my muscles are definitely not ready to do much. So please pray that I have wisdom in trying to figure out how much I can push myself without overdoing it.

Sincerely,

Misty

I slept well that night and woke up early the next morning to contractions. For several hours, I was able to doze on and off between contractions. By the time the nurse came in, I was pretty sure that this would be the day!

On Saturdays, an outside chef was brought in, and he cooked us a special breakfast to order. I ordered an omelet with the works, and a big plate of watermelon. The omelet dripped with cheese and I knew I would need the energy for the day ahead of me. I requested a second plate of watermelon and set it aside to eat during labor.

The doctor came in and checked me. I was starting to dilate and he agreed that today was the day. He decided to go ahead and break my water and get things moving. He knew my body was exhausted and couldn't handle too much, and he wanted to make sure I didn't end up laboring all day and into the night.

He broke my water about 11:30 a.m., and my contractions grew stronger. I was moved to a labor/delivery room across the hall. I paced the hall, pausing to hang my arms around Nathan's neck, for him to support me during the contractions. After a few laps down the hall, I was exhausted. I knew I couldn't handle any more.

We headed back to the room, where I discovered the wonders of a birth ball. It was such a comfortable position to sit on the ball and rock my hips, and I lowered the bed to enable me to rest my head on the bed.

I began to feel panicked and overwhelmed. My weakness enveloped me and I felt like I couldn't stay in control. I had flashbacks of previous labors. I felt like waves of the sea were crashing over me, and I was unable to ride them. Each contraction felt like it left me drowning.

I hollered through each contraction and moaned in between. The nurse came in and checked me, and said I was at four centimeters.

"I can't take this anymore!" I screamed, as the next contraction washed over me.

Nathan tried to comfort me. "Shhh, it's ok. It will just be a few more hours."

I snapped and screamed at him, "Don't tell me to be quiet!!!" It was the only time in my life that I had ever yelled at Nathan. I got back into the bed, curled up, and started sobbing. I knew I couldn't handle a few more hours.

Fifteen minutes later, I was holding Lizzie in my arms! My doctor missed the birth. The nurse peeked in to check on me, just as I said I needed to go to the bathroom. Another contraction hit, and the nurse decided she should check me before I went. I tried to kick her away, but then another contraction came, and I started pushing.

The nurse started yelling for another nurse, as she pulled off my pants. She got them off as I was crowning, and she delivered her first baby ever! It was 2:30 in the afternoon, only three hours since they had broken my water.

I picked up Lizzie right away and put her to my breast. She latched on immediately. Lizzie nursed a full thirty minutes before the nurses took her to weigh her and check her over. The doctor arrived in time to stitch me up from where I had torn.

I was moved to a postpartum room and was so happy to have my baby right with me. Nathan took her and lay on the other bed. Soon father and baby were sound asleep.

A few hours later, Nathan's parents arrived with my girls. Everyone was excited to meet Lizzie. Rosy and Gracie were thrilled to have their sister!

Nathan spent the night with me, but he had to leave very early. He had to work that morning and he planned to come back that evening to bring me home!

When Nathan arrived to get me, we found out that the doctor had forgotten to authorize my departure. It took some red tape but we were finally able to get a verbal authorization.

Over six weeks had passed since I arrived at the hospital and I was so glad to come home! It was such a relief!

Lizzie was a champion nurser, both day and night. The first month was hard, due to my weakness and lack of strength. Michelle stayed with us a few more weeks. She worked hard on filling the freezer with pre-made meals before she left. Soon, life settled into a new normal, but the question of whether we should have any more children was burning in our minds.

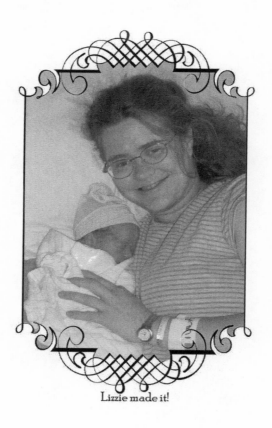

Lizzie made it!

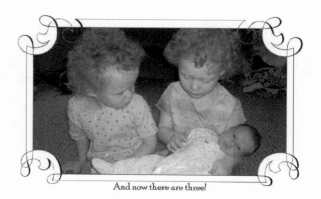

And now there are three!

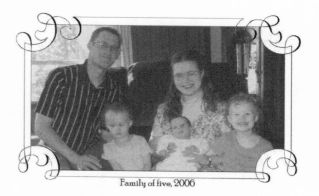

Family of five, 2006

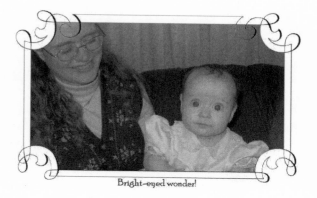

Bright-eyed wonder!

Chapter Eight

But the Lord Directs His Steps

Before Lizzie was born, we had decided that my body needed a break. Now, we wondered if we should even have any more children! We both still believed that children were a blessing from the Lord, and we both still wanted more children. But we had so many questions.

Part of me was willing to sacrifice anything for my children, but the other side asked whether it was right to sacrifice my whole family and my current family for the sake of future children.

Was it right to bring a child into the world, knowing that the risk of preterm labor was so big, and that it could leave them with long-term health issues?

I wanted to teach and train my children, but how could I do that if I was on bed rest? And what about my house? There wouldn't always be a Michelle available to jump in and help me take over. God said women are to be keepers at home. How could I do that if I spent most of my pregnancy on bed rest, and then the next few months recovering? By then, I would likely be pregnant again and repeat the cycle.

We wanted to do God's will. We also wanted to do what was best for our family. Was it time to give up our dreams of having a large family?

The next big question was how we should prevent having more children. I was strongly opposed to hormonal birth control for several reasons. I believe that life begins at conception, and I was not willing to take anything that had even the potential to end a pregnancy.

Even if their purpose was to prevent conception, sometimes that failed. The hormonal birth control could also affect the uterine lining, preventing implantation. I wasn't willing to take that chance, no matter how great or small.

Before I got married, I had stated on more than one occasion, "Abstinence is the only Biblical form of birth control." By now, I had changed my tune.

I had since rethought that opinion and had come to the conclusion that Natural Family Planning with abstinence was NOT a Biblical form of birth control after all. God gives only one reason for abstinence in marriage (excluding purification reasons given in the law), and that is for a time of prayer and fasting mutually agreed upon by both partners.

This didn't leave us many options. We had already seen how effective barrier methods were. We never imagined that we would ever consider any form of permanent birth control, but here we were.

I studied through all the different options. I read all of the various reviews online. As long as I was researching, which was the best permanent option, I didn't have to think about the "if we should" aspect. Finally, we decided that if we were going to go this route, Nathan would get a vasectomy.

Now that we had narrowed it down to what form, we went back to thinking about whether we should even think about doing this. We went over and over all our reasons. We reevaluated our motives, and we sought counsel.

Most people looked at our situation and were confident that this was the best option. A few thought that it could go either way. Only a couple of people were in opposition.

We felt like our hands were tied, and the risks involved with another pregnancy were just too great. Nathan went in to see the doctor. They gave him all the prep info and set a date. It was a done deal--or so we thought.

We fretted about this decision until two days before the appointment. It felt like this should be the right decision, but we just didn't have peace. Finally, we called and canceled the appointment. We were back at square one.

We knew that God is sovereign, and we knew that God wouldn't give us a life that He didn't want us to have. So, we decided to do our part the best we could and pray that God would give us the break we that felt that I needed.

In my mind, the door wasn't closed on the vasectomy option, but this was too serious to step into it without complete confidence that it was the right decision. We went back to using barrier methods and life continued.

When Lizzie was just a few months old, God sent our life into another new direction. We had been praying about a way for Nathan to receive more discipleship and ministry training, and God opened the door.

We decided to move to Phoenix, Arizona to attend Heritage Baptist Church. God provided a job and a house and we were soon on our way.

Having three children, ages three and under, I had felt like one of the bigger families in our church in Colorado. Suddenly, I was one of the smaller ones. The church opened their arms and welcomed us. They taught from the pulpit that children were a heritage from the Lord. I agreed wholeheartedly, but wondered what they would think if they knew our struggle.

I was content to leave things as they were, for now. I knew that someday I would get the itch for another baby, but I was happy with the three that I had. We were starting out with a new house, and I felt as though we were getting a fresh start. I wanted to get back on my feet.

Nathan, however, wrestled with the decisions that we had made. "Will you trust me?" Nathan asked quietly one day. "Will you trust God?"

The questions felt so overwhelming. I knew what he was asking, and I had an idea of the ramifications, though so much was still unknown. Yet again, I was faced with the choice. Was I willing to follow, or was I not? "I will trust," I whispered.

A couple of weeks later, I lay in bed, pondering the verse about man planning his way, but the Lord directing his path. I went and took a pregnancy test, confident that it would be positive. But it wasn't!

I took another test, and another, and yet another. "It is a good thing I got fifty of these tests in bulk," I laughed to Nathan. "Otherwise we would go broke keeping me supplied."

Days went by and pretty soon I was a full week late. "If I am not pregnant, then I am going insane," I ranted. "I have a whole list of symptoms, but the tests just keep showing negative."

Nathan broke out into song, "Have patience, have patience, don't be in such a hurr ..." I tackled him and started tickling him before he could finish the song. Pretty soon, however, I was the one screaming for mercy!

The days dragged on, and my pack of tests dwindled. Test after test showed only one line. By the time I was eleven days late, I was getting frustrated. I hated being in limbo. I had been nauseous for a week, and I was so exhausted. I was sure that I was pregnant.

My emotions were in turmoil. Part of me didn't want to face pregnancy, but part of me was getting excited. I didn't want to admit it, but deep in my heart I was happy, and every negative test was a disappointment!

I skipped a day a day of testing and, the next morning, I took my test, set it on the counter, and walked out. A while later, I remembered that I had forgotten to check the test.

I said goodbye to Nathan, who was heading out the door for his ministry training class. By this time I was tired of the letdown, but I headed back towards the bathroom. I glanced at the test and my eyes widened in surprise! There were clearly two lines!

Since so long had passed since I took it, I had to do another. I watched as the ink inched up the test. Within thirty seconds I had the answer: positive! I danced for joy and quickly called Nathan with the news.

The girls' reaction to having a new baby was so funny. The first thing Rosy said was, "We will have to see whose hair it matches." Gracie cried because she wanted a baby in her tummy, too. That night she cried because she had to go to bed and the baby wasn't here yet.

The pregnancy I had so feared was a reality and I couldn't stop smiling. I was due on September 4, only fifteen months after Lizzie's birthday.

Once the excitement wore off, reality set in. I needed to start looking into caregiver options. I found a place that used both doctors and nurse midwives. The birth would be in the hospital, but I could have some of the benefits of a midwife birth. It seemed as though it could be the best of both worlds.

I enjoyed my first few appointments. I had the chance to meet several of the doctors and midwives, and everything looked perfect. I wondered if I would have a normal pregnancy this time.

I prayed and prayed that God would grant that one request! I thought that God must have been testing me to see if I would be faithful during the previous challenging pregnancies, and I was. I felt that I had passed the test, and now God was going to reward me. I set aside my fears of preterm labor and was confident that all would go smoothly this time!

But things don't always go as we assume, and soon enough I started getting some familiar twinges. My heart sank. I fought the possibility that this could be preterm labor. I was sure that God would not put me through this again.

But there was no question--we were dealing with preterm labor. I made an appointment and ended up with a new doctor. I was only fourteen weeks, and I explained to him my history and told him that I had put myself on bed rest.

"No, no," the doctor shook his head. "Don't start bed rest. The fetus is not viable. You need to get up and let the inevitable happen."

First, I was shocked. Then, I was furious. How could this man have such an utter disregard for life? When we got home, I went straight back on bed rest. I was going to do whatever it took to protect my baby.

I called the office and made another appointment. I told them that I was not willing to see that doctor anymore and I wanted an appointment with either the doctor I had seen previously or with one of the midwives.

Meanwhile, I struggled through my emotions about it not being fair that God would put me through preterm labor again. The question echoed through my mind, "Will you trust me?"

Yet again, I was faced with the very same question. Last time I said yes, God gave me another baby. It was not what I thought I wanted, but I quickly realized that God knew so much better than me. Once again I said, "Yes, God."

We decided that I should keep going to church for a while. Friends donated a recliner so that, once I arrived, I could keep my feet up and my head back. That earned me a lot of attention! People would bow to me, saying, "Yes, Madam, whatever you say, Madam" and would run to get whatever I might need.

Our church rallied around me. Michelle told me that she would love to come again, but she couldn't get away for six weeks. Over the next four weeks, a different family from the church came over each workday. They surrounded me with so much love and support.

Next, a dear friend, Kari, came to visit for a couple of weeks. It was such a pleasure to have her with us. She made it her goal to spoil and pamper me, and she did a good job! The kids quickly dubbed her, "Aunt Kari.

I kept working hard to do the natural remedies that I knew could help prevent preterm labor. I drank tons of water. My goal was a gallon per day, and sometimes I felt like I was going to drown myself. My herbal tinctures helped a ton, but eventually, they just weren't enough.

"I think you should consider taking progesterone shots," my doctor commented.

"Shots???" I replied in surprise. "Aren't there easier ways of getting progesterone? I don't exactly like needles...."

My fear of needles wasn't able to override what the doctor felt best. By the time I left, I was set up to receive progesterone injections twice a week. I felt sick at the thought. Not only did I despise needles, I didn't see how in the world we could pull off two appointments per week!

Thoughts rushed through my head: "How could Nathan take off the time to take me? How could we lose that kind of work and pay the gas, too? Wouldn't getting up and down so much defeat the purpose of bed rest? Needles? Please, NO!"

While I was still fretting about the impracticality of this proposition, the doctor whispered to the nurse. She left and returned shortly, handing him some paperwork.

"I think that you will qualify for in-home care," he announced. "Here is all the information that you will need to get it set up."

Immediately I thought of the verse that says, "Be anxious for nothing, but in everything by prayer and supplication, let your request be made known to God" (Philippians 4:6).

Once again, my fretting jumped the gun, when God already had those details all worked out. It took a little red tape and a lot of phone calls, but soon we were able to get it all arranged. A nurse would be coming every Monday and Thursday to "shot me."

That week, we went in for a sonogram. I suspected that we would have a boy, but since I had thought that last time, I didn't trust my judgment. This time, however, the baby decided to make it very clear that he was a boy!

We were ecstatic! On the way home we started talking about names. For the first time, we didn't name our baby on the way home from the sonogram. We weren't able to agree on a name, so there would still be much discussion.

Rosy told me that of course it was a boy – she'd told me that all along. Gracie pronounced, "It is a boy, a baby, and a brother."

When the nurse arrived for the progesterone shot, she pulled out the biggest needle I had ever seen, and I felt faint. She explained that the progesterone was suspended in very thick oil, so that the absorption would be delayed. This allowed my body to slowly assimilate it over days. By the time it was done, it would be time to get the next shot.

The nurse tried to prep me. "This needle is really hard to get in," she explained as she pulled her arm back as if she were going to pitch a baseball. She thrust the needle into my hip with all her effort. I screamed. It was worse than I expected.

Once the needle was in, she paused to allow me to relax and to describe how the shot would work. Because the

114

liquid was so thick, she had to inject it very slowly. She would inject a little, pull the needle out a little and reinsert it in another spot and inject some more. She repeated the cycle many times.

By the time the shot was done, my thigh ached fiercely. It throbbed excruciatingly for the next twenty-four hours. The nurse told me that the next week we would do the other side, so each side only got one shot per week.

In the beginning, it took the whole week for my hip to feel better. Then it was time for the next shot in the same side. The nurse was very friendly and always blew up gloves into balloons for the girls. They eagerly anticipated each visit, while I dreaded them.

Meanwhile, the name discussion continued. "Ok," Nathan conceded, "We will name him Andrew." I cheered because Andrew was my top pick.

"And will he be Andrew Lansdon?" I asked. Lansdon was my great-grandfather's name, and my grandma really wanted a grand/great grandson to carry on the legacy. I really wanted to do that for her and was thrilled that Nathan agreed.

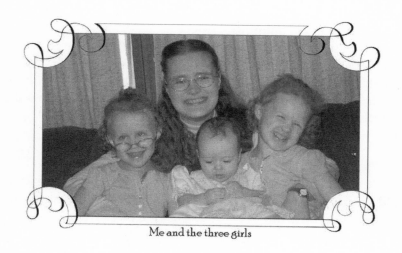

Me and the three girls

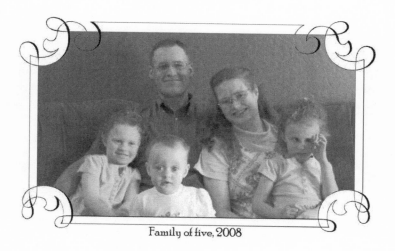

Family of five, 2008

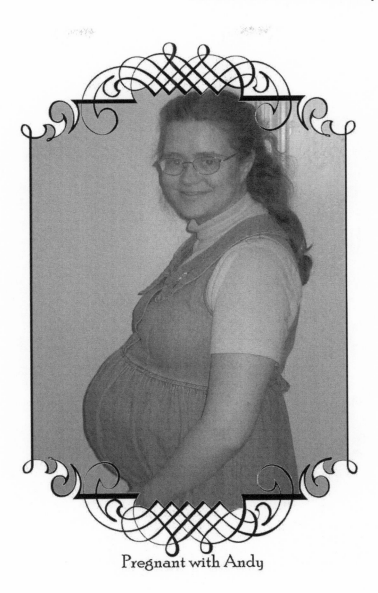

Pregnant with Andy

Chapter Nine

What Time I Am Afraid

We headed to the airport to pick up Michelle! Everyone was excited to see her and we were grateful that she was willing to come in and live with us during this time of need.

Michelle would be staying for the remainder of our pregnancy, so we strove to make life as normal as we could, as we got the girls back into a routine.

Lizzie's first birthday came around. I was already five and a half months pregnant and had been on bed rest for twelve weeks. The rest of the pregnancy loomed ahead, and I knew that it would be a challenging few months.

My sonograms showed that my cervix was shortening slightly. The doctors decided that I should come in every other week to check for more changes. Now that Michelle was here, appointments were so much easier!

The progesterone was leaving me with nasty headaches, and my whole body began to ache. The months of bed rest were starting to take its toll and I could feel my physical strength ebbing away.

As I lay in bed anticipating the end of this pregnancy, it hit me that I could not end the pregnancy without having another labor. Somehow, in the middle of the excitement of a baby and the complications of the pregnancy, I had forgotten about labor.

Fear set in and I felt sick. I started to panic about the thought of going through yet another labor. My heart was pounding, and I cried. Nathan held me in his arms and sang to me. I relaxed and slept.

God was so faithful during these trials. When the discouragement of the pain and weakness and fear were starting to set in, I came across a quote on a friend's blog.

"And yet, it's during these times that we learn our best lessons. When God becomes a close friend and very real. When we learn that we can't 'do it all,' neither should we try. When we realize we're not as invincible as we thought we were, nor do we know as much as we thought we did. When we know for sure that nothing depends on us, but on us depending upon HIM!

"As hard as it is, I will embrace this time. And although, to be honest, I'd rather not be in this place right now, it's where God has me. By His grace, I will walk through, knowing my Best Friend is right beside me, guiding me, holding my hand every step of the way."

This blog post was an inspiration to me. I struggled at times, but this described my heart. I would go back to the post and read it regularly, and it would remind me to keep my trust in God.

Michelle left for two weeks to be with her family. My dad came to visit, and then Nathan's twelve-year-old sister, Evie, came and stayed with us for a week. Everybody was thrilled to have family visits!

One night I got up to go to the bathroom and I lost my balance and fell. The next morning I wrote a friend, "Can you pray for me? I have been having more contractions today, and it seems to be getting worse, not better. I've done two different tinctures, and I will be doing the salt soon. My lower back pressure is increasing, too."

Fortunately, the salts did the trick and we were able to halt the labor ... again.

On July 3, 2008, I sent an email update with our family news:

Dear Family and Friends,

In my last update, I announced that we were having a boy. His name is officially Andrew Lansdon Marr. Or "Little Andy" as his sisters call him.

Andy is still staying where he belongs, despite his frequent attempts to be born. The time is rapidly approaching, and we have decided that in about three weeks we will stop preventing his birth and let him come.

I have been on bed rest for five months now. We are so grateful for Michelle, who has been living with us for several months now. She is keeping things running smoothly around here, and enabling Andy to stay where he belongs.

121

I am having a pretty challenging time, physically. I am pretty much unable to do anything, except to get up for the bathroom. Not only do most forms of movement cause my contractions to start up, my muscles are so weakened, that I can barely do anything if I wanted to. I am out of breath when I roll over in bed, and getting up to go to the bathroom takes every bit of strength that I have.

So, I would appreciate your prayers as we go through these last weeks. Please pray that God will continue to give me the needed grace, and that I will have the strength needed to get through the labor and delivery. Also that He will grant me a speedy recovery.

Nathan has done a great job jumping in and doing many of the things that I feel like I should be doing. And he always does it cheerfully, even though he gets up at 3:30 in the morning for work. I am grateful for his loving support for me right now. He is the best husband a woman could ever hope for!

We have mentioned before that Gracie has Trigger Thumb. After many appointments and a lot of red tape, she finally has surgery scheduled. She will be having it done this Friday. The surgery is relatively minor, but it will be done under a general anesthetic. We'd appreciate your prayers for her safety. Most likely, she will think that the worst part is the no food or drink before the surgery, which will be at 2:30.

Rosy is looking forward to having a brother. She walks around with her doll under her shirt, and talks about when she will be a Mommy. She has been asking me how long it will be until we have eleven children! She is also anxious to start reading and has been working on writing and sounding out letters.

Lizzie is our sweetheart. She is running around, and is trying to talk more and more. She loves to cuddle and is a real charmer. There isn't much that she loves more than for someone to smile at her. And if she is not hungry or tired, then she is usually making us smile. She loves her baby dolls and usually wants Nathan and me to hug and kiss them, too. I think that she will be thrilled to have a new baby!

Please pray that God will give us wisdom in some upcoming decisions. We have to be out of our house by the end of October. We have been praying about where we should go, whether in the same area or closer to Nathan's work. We are praying to find a place for a good bit cheaper. Please pray that God will direct Nathan as he is seeking God's will for us.

My progesterone shots continued biweekly. Rather than my body getting accustomed to them, they became worse and worse. My hips throbbed continuously, making it impossible to get comfortable in any position. Pain was my constant companion.

My doctor wanted me to wait until thirty-seven weeks to stop the shots. Since boys' lungs take longer to develop, they wanted to be sure he was ready!

About a week later, on August 19, the contractions picked up. Pretty soon they were consistent and coming every two to three minutes. As we left for the hospital, an email was sent announcing that the Marr baby was on his way.

As we arrived at the hospital, the fear set in again, and I panicked. After hours of labor contractions, they completely stopped! We went ahead and went in, thinking they would pick back up, but they didn't.

The nurse put the monitor on my stomach, and we watched a flat line. She was irritated with me for wasting her time and said, "You don't know what real labor is. When it starts, you will know it is real."

When she left, I turned to Nathan, "Take me home. I don't want to stay here." We left, and as soon as we pulled away, I had another contraction.

I continued having contractions semi-regularly, but not enough to be considered full labor. Six days later, labor picked back up. This time it was a sure thing--or so we thought. No sooner had we got to the hospital, then labor stopped once again.

My due date was getting closer and I was frustrated. After spending six months on bed rest, why wouldn't this baby just come? Labor would come and go. Whenever I would start to question whether it was time to go to the hospital, the fear would set in and labor would stop. Time inched by.

On August 5, I had an appointment with the nurse midwife who would be delivering me at the hospital. I waited and waited, but she had been called away to a birth. After we had been there several hours, they sent us home. I was disappointed that I wasn't able to discuss my last-minute concerns.

My due date came and went, but no baby yet! I was frustrated with the dread of labor being prolonged. Plus, our moving date was just over three weeks away, and Michelle had a plane ticket in less than two weeks. The plan had been for her to be with us a month after birth. With my other births being thirty-seven, thirty-one, and thirty-seven weeks, plus having preterm labor, we never expected to go full term!

The contractions continued to come and go, teasing me with the possibility of labor, and flirting away. I'd finally had enough. Time to pull out the castor oil!

At 5:00 a.m., the morning of September 10, I made myself a chocolate milkshake. I used vanilla ice cream as the base, added a generous amount of chocolate syrup, and poured in the castor oil. I tested it, gagged, and immediately doubled the amount of chocolate.

Though masked with chocolate, the taste of the castor oil brought back a flood of memories of Rosy's labor. I felt sick with the thought of going through labor again. Soon, that wasn't the only type of sickness I felt.

I went back to bed, hoping to sleep off the first few hours and wake up in labor. My plans were thwarted, as I lay in bed, moaning and groaning with terrible stomach cramps.

"How could I have done this to myself?" I moaned. I had no one to blame but myself, and blame myself I did!

I was too sick to even fret about labor. I stayed curled up moaning for five hours, and then finally the misery lifted. After that, the contractions started picking up, and I knew the end was soon--though it wasn't as soon as I expected.

We knew we didn't want this labor to stop, so we were proactive in keeping the contractions going. I pulled out the breast pump, and Michelle helped "rub up contractions." She did a circular massage on my stomach that would bring on a contraction every time. We also tried massaging pressure points.

Labor kept picking up steadily, and we finally headed out to the hospital for the third time. "This has to be it," I commented dryly, "'cause three strikes and you're out."

I noticed the people milling around the waiting area. Just like the other two visits, contractions were letting up. The nurses said that they were too busy to check me yet, and told me to either wait in the hall or come back later.

I wasn't about to leave, so we started pacing the halls. We went round and round the corridor, and the contractions were picking back up. I was pretty sure we were annoying some of the workers, and it made me nervous. Nathan told me to just ignore them, and we kept walking.

Eventually, someone came out and told me to stop walking, so I wouldn't end up having the baby before they had a room ready. "You can't have the baby yet," they explained. "We need to get another lady dispatched and the room cleaned. Just sit down, relax, and wait."

"I want to have this baby NOW," I told Nathan, "just to show them that I can." Nathan laughed and told me that I was obviously close to birth; otherwise I would have been much more compliant.

I was finally ushered back. They confirmed this was indeed labor and admitted me to my room. They asked for my midwife's phone number and promised to call her.

The nurse handed me a little gown and told me to put it on. "My midwife told me that it would be OK for me to wear my own clothes. Would that be a problem?"

"Yes," she huffed. "You have to wear this." And she put the gown into my hands.

I realized this was probably the first of many battles, and I decided this wasn't a battle to die on. I heard that the doctor who had told me to not go on bed rest and to "let the inevitable happen" was on call for the next few hours. "Do not let him come in here," I told Nathan. "I'm serious. I do not want him to even walk in this room."

I assumed that my nurse midwife would get there any minute, and I wouldn't have to worry about the doctor. I was exhausted from all my pacing the halls and was relieved to find a birth ball. I sat on the ball next to the bed and asked Nathan to adjust the height of the bed, so that I could rest my head.

The contractions were really picking up, and I was feeling more stressed about my midwife not being there. "Can I come in?" a voice called from the doorway. A lady walked in the room.

"Hi, I am the nurse midwife on call," she explained. "They have tried to get in touch with your midwife, but they couldn't get through to her."

My emotions were so mixed. I wanted my nurse midwife, but I was so relieved to have someone with me, so the doctor on call wouldn't feel the need to check on me. I would be more relieved when he was gone.

Labor was full blown and we knew the end was getting close. The fear was setting in again and I wasn't handling the labor very well.

"Why don't you try another position?" the nurse midwife asked me. I couldn't think of any other positions. She tried to explain what she wanted me to do, but I couldn't understand. I started crying and she backed off. I really wanted her to help me and show me what she meant, but she was so hands off that she just went back to her seat and left me to deal with it on my own.

Finally, Nathan suggested that I get on the bed, and the midwife checked me. "You can push whenever you feel the urge," she informed me.

The clock read 11:25 p.m. and I turned to Nathan and said, "His birthday will be September 10." I was wrong.

As I pushed with the contractions, I knew something was wrong. He just wasn't budging. I pushed for over one and a half hours. The nurse midwife was very hands off, but later she told me that his head was tilted to the side. Because of that tilt, I tore internally before he crowned and I had to push him through excruciating pain.

Finally, at 1:05 a.m. on September 11, Andy was born! It was instant love! However, I had been up since 5:00 a.m. I had only slept three hours the night before, and I was exhausted. The midwife worked on stitching me up, while the nurses took Andy to weigh and clean up.

The stitches seemed to take forever. "How many stitches have you done?" I asked.

"I don't know," the midwife replied. "I forgot to count. You tore almost all the way through."

I later learned that the tear and long pushing time could have been easily prevented. Had the midwife straightened his head while still in the birth canal, Andy would have likely had his September 10 birthday, and my recovery would have been much less painful.

Andy nursed beautifully! I was so relieved to have my baby in my arms and the labor behind me. I thought back over my pregnancy, and so many aspects seemed hellish. But two things were clear.

First, God had been faithful! He carried us through the entire way, providing for all the specifics and using His people to shower us with love.

Second, it had been worth it! I looked down at the little face nestled in my arms and my heart melted. God had given me a son, and I would never regret that. The trials were but for a moment in comparison to the life of my little boy. God knew that I needed Andy so much more than I needed a break. And I praised Him.

Michelle left ten days after Andy was born and we prepared to move. My body was pretty weak and worn, but I didn't see how I could possibly stay down and recover. We had to be out of our house just ten days later.

My mom came to visit us, bringing my little sisters, one only months older than Andy! People rallied around us and somehow we got the work done. Soon we were settled into our new house. I was starting to get back on my feet, but the pregnancy complications weren't over yet.

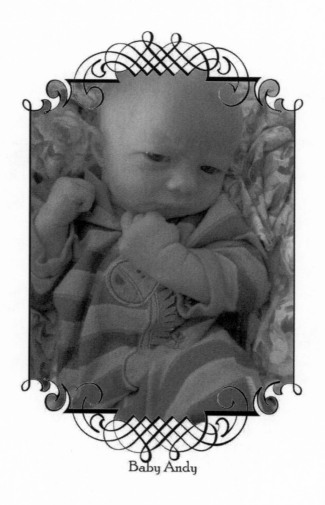

Baby Andy

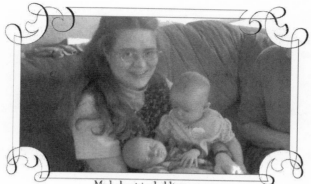

My baby sister holding my son

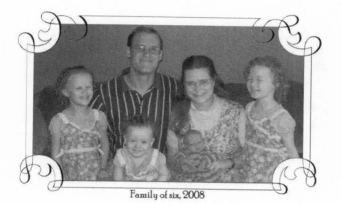

Family of six, 2008

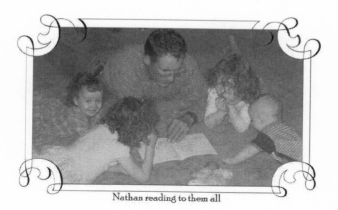

Nathan reading to them all

Chapter Ten

Even in the Valley

When Andy was about three months old, my progesterone levels dropped abruptly. Because the progesterone shots create such an abnormal high in my body, the drop was also extreme. When my progesterone level plummeted, post-partum depression set in.

Overnight I went from cheerful and encouraged to wallowing in the depths of despair. I have always been a "glass half full" kind of a person, and even when I did struggle in the midst of a challenge, I had learned to push through it and be joyful. But this was different!

There were no extenuating circumstances that were troubling me this time. Yet it felt as though there was a cloud of doom hanging over me and I couldn't shake it. I felt like I hated life, and I hated myself for feeling like that. My mind knew that it wasn't so, but I felt trapped in a dysfunctional body.

"Yes, you can watch the movie again," I sighed, and rolled over on the couch. The DVD player had become my babysitter. I hated it, but it kept my kids together, in my line of vision.

Nathan was a rock that held my life together. He loved me through the pain. When I felt tempted to end everything, it was his love for me that held me back from making foolish choices. He deserved better.

Though it felt like an eternity, this went on for a month. I realized that I needed help. I finally reached out to a friend. She and another friend came over and cleaned my house. She also contacted Lisa, another friend who knows so much about treating things naturally.

Lisa came up with a plan for me. She had me use a natural progesterone cream, told me to take a couple fatty supplements (cod liver oil and Omega 3-6), and to add coconut oil to my diet. During this time, we had been eating quite frugally, and were consuming very little fats and produce.

The fog started lifting within twenty-four hours, and it was pretty much gone in three days. I was amazed! The physical transformation was so astounding. I couldn't believe just how much benefit those few changes made! I loved life again, and I was ready to press forward and conquer this challenge.

I was not home free yet. If I delayed a dose of progesterone cream, the fog would start to show itself. With four children, ages five and under, it was easy to forget. Nathan left early, but he would call me from work every day to make sure I used my cream. If I hadn't remembered, he had me use it while on the phone to confirm that I didn't forget.

Months went by and the struggle against the depression reduced. As my body adjusted to balancing its own hormones, I was able to gradually reduce and eventually eliminate the progesterone. I was grateful to God for His mercy to me in helping us come up with a solution.

About this time, I got pregnant again. I was not expecting a pregnancy so soon, and it took me by surprise. I was scared of having another little one so close and concerned about all my body had gone through. I was still working through those emotions when we lost the baby. On one side I was sad, but I also felt relief. Since we hadn't announced the pregnancy, once again I decided not to tell anyone. I knew I would feel guilty by those who expected me to be grieving more, and I knew there would be some who would think it was best.

I didn't want to deal with either side ... so I didn't.

"What can we do to reduce living expenses?" Nathan asked me. "Surely there has to be a way to live cheaper than we are living now." We had already figured out that we really shouldn't cut the grocery budget any more, and we spent little more than the basic bills.

We brainstormed ideas and talked about RVs. We got enthusiastic about that option, but couldn't figure out a way to make it realistic. Eventually, we landed on the idea of a mobile home.

Meanwhile, I got pregnant again. This time I felt more ready and we rejoiced at the news! It complicated the idea of moving a little, so we decided we'd better push through now. We wanted to be settled before there was any risk of preterm labor.

LESSONS LEARNED

We found a small two-bedroom mobile home at a good price. The rent for the plot and payment for this home would cut hundreds of dollars a month from what we were paying for rent.

Thus began the flurry of reducing our stuff, having yard sales, selling on EBay, and packing. It felt like a fun challenge to see what we could get rid of, and how much money we could get from it. We were able to cover the moving costs from the money we earned. Eleven months after we had moved into this house, we left.

Our church jumped in and helped us move. Then my family came to visit and helped with little details that would make the house more efficient. My mom took me to Sam's Club and filled my freezer full of frozen dinners.

For such a small trailer, the layout was great. There was a bedroom on each end, while the living room, dining room and kitchen were one big open room in between. It made the space feel bigger and more comfortable.

The first midwife I met was not willing to take me as a patient. "You are too high risk," she told me. "I will only take you if you see a specialist simultaneously. If you reach thirty-six weeks, you can drop the specialist and use me exclusively."

Using and paying for two different caregivers wasn't an option, so I kept looking.

I finally found a midwife, Pam White, who was willing to work with me. We wanted to hopefully prevent preterm labor, or at least treat it more naturally. After two emergency hospital births, and two planned home births, we were once again shooting for a home birth!

136

My first visit with Pam reminded me just how much I preferred going with a home birth midwife, rather than through a more conventional hospital route. With Pam, I felt like an individual, not a statistic. I appreciated that Pam was open to hearing my story and working with me on how to best prevent, and possibly treat bed rest. Pam agreed that she would do her best to help me have a natural home birth. I agreed that if she felt the need, I would go back to the hospital.

The pregnancy got off to a great start with minimal morning sickness. I was hopeful that things might be different this time, but it wasn't long before I felt some cramping. "Well, looks like I will be back on bed rest within a week," I told Nathan. "This is how it always starts. But this time it is earlier than ever."

I doubled up on all of my preterm labor tricks. I took my tinctures, soaked in Epsom salts, drank my water, and ate more protein. A week went by and I was pleased to see that things were different this time after all. The cramping continued on and off, but it didn't turn into full contractions for nearly two more months!

All my efforts paid off and saved me from being completely down. During that time, I just had to be careful not to overexert myself, and I was able to maintain a relatively normal life.

Unfortunately, the preterm labor eventually came. Once again, I was on bed rest. This time I had very little help. No one was able to come to stay with us. While church friends popped in a couple times a week to lend a hand, most of the time, I was on my own. Our open room was perfect to keep the kids within earshot.

Rosy was now five years old and she was my right hand helper. She was proud that I could count on her! She became an expert cheese toast and peanut butter sandwich maker. The kids ate these two items for breakfast and lunch almost every day! I didn't know how else to handle things, so I ate freezer meals almost every day.

"I'm home!" Nathan announced as he walked in the door after work. "It's so good to see you," he told me as he hugged me. "What should I make for supper tonight?"

On the weekends, Nathan would cook a big pot of beans, so we could eat those several nights a week. The rest of the days, we depended on the freezer food my mom had given us.

Because Rosy and the kids had an extra load to carry, I decided to make it fun. We ordered a giant bag of Yummy Earth Organic suckers. When there were chores to do, I would count, while the kids would run around and see how much they could do before I finished.

Once we got the job done, the kids each got a sucker! Since these were healthier than normal candy, I didn't mind giving them several per day. The kids would regularly come to me and ask if they could do a job to earn a sucker.

The weeks dragged on. My days were spent on the couch, directing the children and trying to keep them productive. Not much happened as long as I stayed down and did everything I was supposed to do. I often had regular contractions, but I was able to either keep them from turning into full labor, or I was able to stop the labor before it picked up too much.

Pam kept a close watch on me and checked me to see if I was dilating. We felt that we had a handle on the preterm labor and that there was no need to see a doctor or add any prescription medications.

I was growing fast. I felt like I was so much bigger than before. I pulled out old pregnancy pictures from previous pregnancies and compared them. I was bigger--a lot bigger!

"I really want you to have sextuplets," Rosy announced, "But I would be happy if it is just twins."

Just twins? I didn't tell Rosy, but I was beginning to suspect that this really was twins. As the weeks went by, I kept growing and I felt more and more confident that we were having twins.

Finally, we decided to go ahead and get a sonogram. Money was an issue, but after calling around, we found a school that would do them for free. In exchange for the free sonogram, we had to allow a student in the room, and the tech would explain every detail of the sonogram to the student.

We were excited about this sonogram, and I was looking forward to the play-by-play account. But I was even more excited about finding out how many babies there were.

We arrived at the school and they ushered us all back. They were friendly and welcomed the kids, and were quick to explain to them what was happening. It was clear very quickly that there was just one baby. I felt a twinge of disappointment that there weren't two.

After a few minutes, our baby decided to make things obvious.

"Do we have a Rebekah Faith Marr?" I grinned and asked Nathan.

"It looks like we do," he responded. "And it looks like the girls win four to one."

After having had Michelle with us the past two pregnancies, we all missed her this time around. We were excited to find out that she was going to be flying through Tucson, Arizona, and would have some time there. We decided to head out that way and see her. It was great to visit with her for a little while, even though she wasn't able to stay long. We visited for a few hours and then headed back home.

"Ouch," I cried out, as I tried to get to the bathroom. My sciatic nerve was acting up and it would randomly freeze up. "Please help me," I shook Nathan to wake him. "I can't get up." Once I was on my feet I could get myself to the bathroom, but this scene happened almost every night, often several times in one night.

Because of the pain from moving, I was getting very little sleep. Often it was only two to three hours a night. I was having a harder time coping during the day.

As I grew bigger Bekah's head was pressing hard against my cervix. This exacerbated the pressure and pain, making labor feel more imminent. "What was that?" I wondered as I felt the pressure let up. I put my hand on my tummy and I could feel Rebekah turn. Ahh, instant relief!

But my feeling of relief was short lived. I realized that, while the relief of the pressure felt good, it also meant that my baby was no longer head down and that meant that, if I went into labor, she would be breech.

I went online and read all kinds of stuff about getting babies to turn. However, after talking to Pam, we decided to hold off and see if she would go back on her own. Eventually Bekah did turn head down again. It is amazing how the pressure that once felt annoying was now a relief!

Rebekah decided to spend the next few weeks teasing me. She went head up again, and then back down--several times. Finally, as I was reaching thirty-six weeks, she went down to stay.

Nathan's sister, Evie, came and stayed a few weeks with us towards the end of the pregnancy. We all enjoyed home cooking again, and the kids were thrilled to have someone to take them outside for some fresh air!

When I hit thirty-six weeks, I got up from bed rest, and we fully expected Bekah to be born right away. But Bekah continued to tease us--this time with on and off labor. We called my midwife, Pam, several times, but didn't quite reach the point of having her come.

I was weak and felt very fragile. I could get around, but I was not strong enough to do much of anything. I was concerned about the approaching labor. Part of me fretted that it would be just as bad as my previous births, but this time I would be having a home birth, and a water birth at that!

My midwife was aware of my concerns and we were able to talk about my expectations and hopes for this labor. I knew that she would be working with me to help me achieve it!

My mom and little sisters arrived. They had hoped to get here in time for the birth, but little did we know that they would barely make the birth before they had to leave! My due date came and went, and we went in to see Pam. We finally decided to have my membranes stripped, but still no labor.

Finally, a week past my due date, I woke up to a strong contraction. By the time it was time for Nathan to leave for work, I had had several contractions. "Please don't leave me!" I cried with my arms around his neck. He held me as another contraction came on. "I don't want you to miss work," I fussed. "You really need to go. You can't stay here and just hope today is the day."

Nathan chuckled at my mixed messages. "I am not going anywhere," he assured me.

"But ..." I started to protest. Nathan interrupted my protest with a kiss. I pulled away to breathe through another contraction. "Thank you," I responded. "I really need you here."

As the morning wore on, the contractions picked up. Nathan called Pam and two other friends--Lisa and Christina--who planned to be at my birth. Once they got there, my contractions stalled out.

Pam sent Nathan out to walk me around the neighborhood. As we walked, the contractions picked back up. But no sooner than we got back home, they puttered out again.

"You look exhausted," Pam commented. "What you really need is a nap." Pam, Lisa, and Christina left and I went to bed. I felt frustrated to go through all those contractions only to end in nothing.

I fell asleep and slept soundly for two hours. Once again, I awoke to a contraction. This one was my strongest one yet! It was quickly followed by another, and another. Nathan called Pam, Lisa, and Christina to come back and started filling up the birth pool.

Pretty soon, it was clear that birth was imminent and I was ready to get in the pool. As the contractions increased, I started to panic. Lisa took my hand and told me to breathe. "I don't know how," I cried, as fear set in.

Nathan sat just out of the pool and held my shoulders. Lisa walked me through how to relax and breathe through the contractions. With each contraction, I would start to panic and Lisa would walk me through when to breathe in, when to breathe out. I felt my body relax, and I got though the contraction without tensing up.

But as soon as the next contraction came, I reverted to the old habits, and Lisa would walk me through how to respond to the contraction. She told me exactly how to respond to the contraction over and over and over.

The water around me was also conducive to relaxing. As the contractions would hit, I would lift my body and float. Nathan kept his arms under my arms, so I didn't have to worry about going under water. While I was floating, I wasn't able to brace my arms or legs against the side, and that helped to keep my body relaxed.

I began to get in a rhythm. I stayed in the reclining back position for several hours, with Nathan holding me up and Lisa guiding me through each contraction. This labor was so vastly different than my previous labors! By this point, I would have been thrashing and screaming, but I was in complete control and had not screamed even once.

Lisa kept me supplied with cool rags for my forehead. They felt so good, and I was always ready for the next one. Then, suddenly it didn't feel good. I didn't want that thing on me. Lisa started to put the next one on my forehead and I slapped her hand away.

It was clear that the end was near, and I got on my knees to push. I faced out leaning on the edge of the tub and holding onto Nathan. "This is it, Misty. Push now," Pam instructed. I pushed with all my might but the contraction ended before she was born. As the next contraction hit, I pushed again, and I cried out with my first scream in the labor.

"Grab her, Nathan, grab her," I heard Pam saying to Nathan. I realized that Rebekah had been born! Just like that! Since I was on my knees and Nathan was in front of me, Pam wanted Nathan to grab Bekah and pull her up towards the front of me, so that I could sit down. He put Bekah into my arms as I sank back into the water. I held Bekah on my shoulder, so that her head would be above water.

"My baby, oh my baby," I murmured as I kissed her soft cheeks. For the next few minutes, it seemed as though there was no one in the world but me and little Bekah.

What an amazing experience this was! In past births, relief overpowered all other feelings. But now, all I could think of was how much I loved my little one, and how worth it this all was.

My mom called in my kids and little sisters. Everyone came in to peek at Rebekah, and then she ushered them out. They were so excited to see her right after birth!

Eventually, I delivered the placenta and they helped me out of the water to the bed. "Did I tear?" I asked the midwife. I was hoping to avoid that aspect of recovery!

"It looks like just a skid mark," Pam replied. "It's not quite a tear. If you are careful and keep your legs together for a while, I don't think we need to do anything."

I reflected over how many firsts this labor had for me. It was the first time I had the labor/birth I had wanted. It was the first time I didn't panic and allow the fear to take over. It was the first time I didn't scream through the labor. It was the first time I maintained control. It was the first time I was handed my baby and was able to bask in the love without being interrupted by my baby being whisked away. It was my fifth birth, yet so full of firsts!

All of the wonders of the firsts eventually dissipated as this became my most challenging postpartum recovery. It started with Bekah struggling with breathing. It seemed like there was mucus left over from birth. We couldn't get anything out with the nose aspirator, so we assumed that it would work its way out eventually.

That night, I held her in my arms and tried to sleep. Each time I dozed off, I heard the raspy noise of her breathing, and I would wait and make sure she was able to get the breath in. She usually got her breath in fine, just with a lot of noise, but every now and then she had an even harder time and it would wake her, too.

I stayed awake nearly the entire night, with only a little dozing here and there. I was so happy to be able to stay in bed the next day!

"Nathan, Bekah is having a hard time nursing," I said in frustration. "Every time she latches on, she pulls back, trying to breathe."

Over the next few days, nursing got harder. All her on and off latching created cracks and extreme pain. I cried when she latched on, and I cried when she didn't.

"I think that nursing struggles are the most emotional thing ever, for a woman," I informed Nathan. "It feels like it brings into question your ability to be a good mother. Add her breathing issues on top of that, and ..." I burst out crying again.

When Pam came back to check on Bekah and me, she thought that her nasal cavity was a bit swollen. I began reading and researching what could help, deciding to try a humidifier and essential oils. They helped but, for the most part, we just had to wait it out. Pam said that, as Bekah grew, her nasal passage would open a little more and it would no longer be a concern.

146

Bekah was struggling to get enough air in. At this point she was able to breathe, but sounded like she wouldn't be able to keep breathing. Everything we did for her helped enough to ensure that she would get through this OK, but it didn't help me sleep.

For the next several weeks, I only slept in bits and pieces, constantly alert to Bekah, making sure she took that next breath!

"Nathan, you won't believe what I did," I laughed one evening. "I wrote a letter to Lisa and signed it, 'Lisa.' I told you I was tired!"

Meanwhile, the pain from my "skid-mark" wasn't improving. It was getting worse. When I was staying down the first few days, I knew that it hurt, but I expected that. I wasn't expecting it to get much worse as I started to get up.

At first, I was only getting up in little bits. As I started getting up more, the pain increased to the point that I couldn't even stand without doubling over in pain.

"There is something wrong," I informed Nathan. "This is just not right. This is worse than any episiotomy or tear that I have ever had."

We called Pam and decided to go back in to have her check me. Getting in the car and going was excruciating, but I knew that we needed to know what was happening.

"I think I know what the problem is," Pam commented after checking me. "You have a vaginal hematoma. No wonder you are in so much pain!"

LESSONS LEARNED

A hematoma is much like a blood clot/blister. It was caused by trauma in the birth canal as Bekah's head was descending. The hematoma was 3/4 inch in diameter and about two inches long.

Pam explained that ideally the hematoma should resolve on its own; it would just take time. The worst case scenario was that I would need surgery and lancing. We went back home with instructions to stay down and see what happened.

The next few weeks were long and painful. It was stressful dealing with both the hematoma pain and Bekah's breathing challenges. We praised God that within a month the hematoma was resolved and it didn't require any additional intervention.

By the time that I was up and on my feet, Bekah was breathing well. I breathed a sigh of relief to be past this crazy postpartum season. I was ready to move onto the next chapter of my life. Little did I realize how many adventures and changes it would hold!

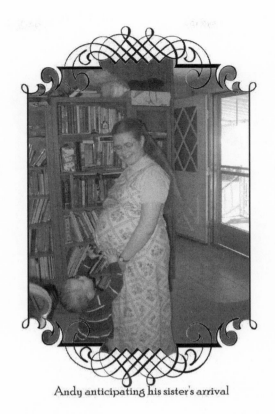

Andy anticipating his sister's arrival

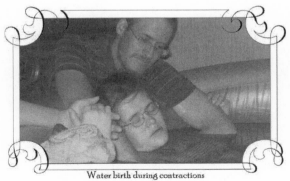

Water birth during contractions

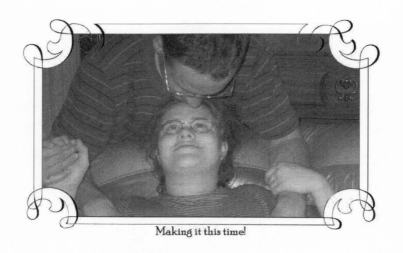

Making it this time!

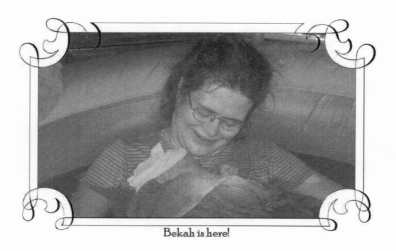

Bekah is here!

Chapter Eleven

Mourning Turned to Joy

"I think we should think about moving," Nathan announced.

"Wha....? Really?" I stuttered. I had resigned myself to being in our tiny mobile home for several years and I didn't think moving was an option.

"Yes," Nathan explained. "The housing market has dropped and I think we can buy a real house with a payment similar to what we are paying here."

I was afraid to get excited, as I didn't want to get my hopes up, just to be disappointed. While I had adjusted to the challenges of the inside of the mobile home, having practically no yard for the kids was a serious disadvantage.

And so we began the house hunt! We read, looked, visited, researched, etc. We found a great realtor. Bridgette had retired from Realty, but had returned to it on a small scale, because she loved it so much. It was clear that she had our best interest in mind, and we felt comfortable, knowing that she would do her best for us.

Pretty soon we found a house that would work for us, but when the offer was put in, someone else offered a cash offer that was higher than the asking price. We were disappointed, but continued the search. We found another house, and no sooner had we put in the offer, we found out that someone else had also put in a higher cash offer.

Thus the cycle continued. Investors had discovered the price drop and the sellers were more interested in the cash than in finding the right family.

I was feeling like this was a never-ending search. The process of agreeing to submit an offer was emotional, and I was tired of the ups and downs of deciding on a house and then being turned down.

"I am tired of this," I told Nathan. "I wish you could go look at the houses by yourself. And if we ever have an offer accepted, THEN you could tell me about the house. I don't even want to see it before then."

"Is that what you really want?" Nathan asked.

"Well, no...." I knew I wanted to have some say in which house we bought. "I am just so done with this."

"It'll all work out," Nathan assured me, as he gave me a squeeze and a peck on my forehead. "Just wait and see."

We left our children with friends and scheduled a viewing for five different houses. As we walked through the first four houses, there was something about each house that just didn't work for me. Normally, I was much more agreeable and willing to work around the dislikes. But not today. I just wasn't interested in those houses.

"At this rate, we won't have to worry about cash offers beating us," Nathan joked.

We headed off to see the fifth house. As we walked through the door into a spacious open room, I knew this was it.

"I want this house," I announced, before I even looked around the rest of the house.

We took the tour and liked what we saw. The house was almost 1600 square feet, three bedrooms, and two baths. It was smaller than many of the houses we looked at, but it was so open that it felt bigger. This was the perfect place for hospitality, and we knew we wanted to be able to have lots of company. The one-acre yard was a big draw as well.

We put in our offer for the house and we heard that there were no other offers. For the first time in a while, we were hopeful that we would actually get this home. And we did!

We breathed a sigh of relief and we rejoiced at the news that we finally had a house!

We went through all the red tape involved in purchasing a new home. Soon, we had the keys in hand.

We packed up and prepared to move. It was so exciting to go from a tiny house with a little shed to a normal house with a garage. I didn't have to do a major decluttering and that made the process so much easier. It wasn't long before we were settled into our new home.

Our kids loved the open space. Bekah showed her approval by learning to walk at nine months, and to run by ten months. She was all over the new house, enjoying the space!

Soon, I began to notice some tell-tale signs and I felt excitement well up. I took a test and it was negative. I tried not to be disappointed. I knew that it really was too early to get a positive, even if I was pregnant.

"Do you think I really am pregnant?" I asked Nathan hopefully.

Nathan hugged me and laughed. "Well, with you," he said, "you never know."

Pretty soon we had an answer. I was indeed pregnant! By now, I was feeling well. Life had settled down into a happy normal, and I was ready for a new baby.

But this pregnancy didn't last long. Within just a few weeks, I lost the baby. I was heartbroken. I had really wanted this little one.

As I grieved the loss of our baby, the memory of my last miscarriage washed over me. I realized that because I hadn't felt ready to be pregnant, I had simply brushed off the death of my baby.

Guilt swept over me, as the reality sunk in. I was mourning one child, yet had felt a twinge of relief with the other. Now I realized that both were equally my children. I imagined what it would be like if I had not had the prior miscarriage. That little one would be a toddler running around my house. Would it have been another girl? Or would Andy have had a brother after all?

In my mind's eye, I pictured the little one running to me, throwing his arms around my neck, exclaiming, "I love you, Momma." I imagined his excitement of having another baby and his sadness about losing this sibling. But it wasn't to be.

I wept. Not only was I grieving the loss of this baby, but I was also grieving the loss of my previous baby. I hugged my pillow and sobbed till there were no tears left. I wrote my mom about some of my emotions over that next week.

June 20, 2011

I am really grieving this loss. ... It is so hard. I am doing pretty well, physically. I'm mostly back to normal, with minimal cramping. We did a lot of sit-on-the-couch school stuff today and that worked out good. I felt productive without having to work too hard.

Emotionally, I'm doing OK. It was pretty rough on me, and I have really grieved this loss. Though I was not very far along, in the 10 days that we did know about the pregnancy (plus another 4-5 days that I suspected), we already felt like he was part of the family. The kids would hug my tummy good night, and were planning new sleeping arrangements. Names were the big discussion every day. And suddenly all those dreams, hopes and plans were all ripped away.

We had prayed for "Junior" during family worship. So, the kids really felt the loss. They had tons of questions, and that was a little hard for me to deal with. But we made it through the roughest part. Things have settled down and we have picked up the pieces and are moving on. Still some occasional tears, but that is to be expected.

June 23, 2011

Last night, Lizzie came and hugged me big. She said, "I am hugging our dead baby. Is it nice to hug our dead baby?" Just 10 minutes later, Andy jumped on me, then stopped and asked, "I not hurt our baby?" Sigh, it is still so hard.

This is my fifth miscarriage. The first three were before any other children, and I grieved over those! Then I had four kids in four years. My fourth miscarriage was when Andy was just a few months old, and I felt like I was drowning. Rather than grieve, I beat myself up with guilt for not wanting the baby. I wrongfully convinced myself that the loss was not as hard because now I had other children.

Now I have five children, and I so wanted this baby! The loss was so hard. It hit me that this loss was not any easier than my first three, and the fact that I had other children didn't make this baby any less valuable. Now I am feeling so sad about not grieving for the baby I lost 2 1/2 years ago. It is like I am grieving that loss for the first time, along with this one.

The next couple of weeks were hard for me, but eventually I knew that it was time to wipe my tears, and pick up and move on. Soon, I was sending another letter!

July 21, 2011

Dear Momma and Daddy,

I wanted to let you know that I am pregnant again! I was surprised that it happened so quickly, and I really wasn't suspecting it this time, but the tests were very clearly positive! Everybody is thrilled, and the kids are already making plans for twins, lol. I am feeling pretty good and have no signs of any problem.

Andy is a little concerned about this, though. He thinks that putting our baby in my tummy is no way to treat our baby. He wants me to get the baby out now. As I grow, he will start to understand better. Bekah obviously doesn't understand, but yesterday she met a new little newborn and was so excited. I think that she will do great! The others are all bouncing for joy, and discussing who will get to take care of the baby. I love hearing their excited enthusiasm.

Misty

The pregnancy started out as all pregnancies start--with exhaustion! I found myself falling asleep at the dinner table or while reading books to the kids. But as the first trimester was winding down, I felt great!

I did have some morning sickness, but not too much and not too long. It stayed within a reasonable time period, and I was OK with that. Before this pregnancy, I had worked hard with changing our diet and eating healthier. I felt like I was seeing a lot of fruit from those changes!

As I watched my body change and my tummy grow, I felt a little nervous, waiting to see what would happen. "Will I have preterm labor again, or will the health changes I made make a difference?" I wondered.

At eighteen weeks, I started feeling movement. It was amazing to be on my feet and active at that point! The time where we have a sonogram was quickly approaching. Up till now, I had never even considered not having a sonogram. A sonogram was a given. Or was it?

Lisa shared with me some of her cautions of sonograms and possible risk factors. As I researched, I learned that there were risks that I had never considered. I did not consider the risk level high, but was it necessary?

After praying and discussing it, we decided that, unless a problem came up, we would skip the sonogram this time. I couldn't believe that I would make a decision like that. I remembered talking to a friend not that long ago. "I would never choose to not find out whether I am having a boy or girl. I couldn't even imagine not knowing." And now, my tune was changing.

I found myself anticipating labor. I had only ever dreaded labor before, but because I had a great birth last time, I now had hope again. I started daydreaming of that moment when I would discover whether this baby was a boy or a girl.

In spite of the anticipation of finding out at labor, I felt something was missing. Many people really start bonding with their baby when they first get a positive pregnancy test result, others when they hear the heartbeat, and yet others when they start to feel movements.

For me, that bonding began when the baby had a name. Up till that moment, I feel excited for my baby, but they become an individual to me once they have a name. Before that, they are an unknown baby; after that, they are themselves. Not naming our baby postponed that feeling and made it harder for the reality of a new baby to sink in.

In the beginning of the second trimester, I decided to take what I had learned about health a little further. We began the GAPS diet. The GAPS diet takes the premise that most illness begins in the gut and that our lack of good gut health prevents our body from dealing with the physical issues that come our way.

The goal of the GAPS diet is to heal our gut lining and nourish our body. Bone broth and fermented foods became a staple in our diet. The GAPS diet only allowed whole foods, and only those that were easy to digest and nourishing to our body.

This was not a "lose weight" diet, nor did it ever restrict calories. If anything, I ate more calories than I ever had. I saw benefits within a few days, and by a few weeks, I felt healthier and stronger than I had in many years. And I felt that while pregnant!

The time frame in which I had grown to expect preterm labor came and went. But my body was still going strong. I was gaining weight, but it was all baby. For the first time, I didn't get puffy and flabby during my pregnancy. I felt good--really good.

During the second trimester I was on my feet and working hard. There was a lot of extra food prep that went along with the GAPS diet, as everything was from scratch. I worked hard to get my house in better order, from all the downtime I had endured. I cleaned, I organized, I sorted. I even stocked the freezer with pre-made meals. And I still felt good.

I continued staying on top of my preterm labor prevention plan, and that was working out great.

One day I had just finished up washing a sink of dishes and was working of tidying the rest of the kitchen. "Momma, Momma," Andy grabbed at my dress and pulled anxiously. "Hurry up! You need to change."

"Why do you think I need to change?" I wondered.

"We don't want to let the baby get wet!"

It was exciting to experience pregnancy on my feet. We were grateful for this season of normal pregnancy life. It was the sixth time I had reached this point in pregnancy, but the first time I was actually on my feet.

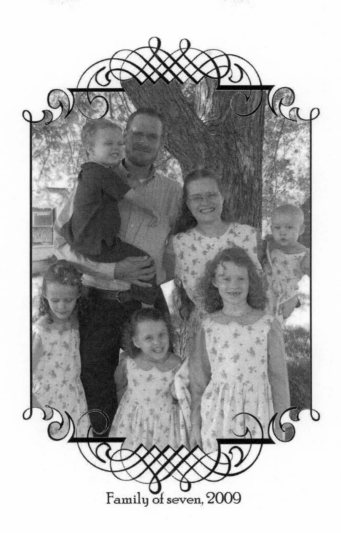

Family of seven, 2009

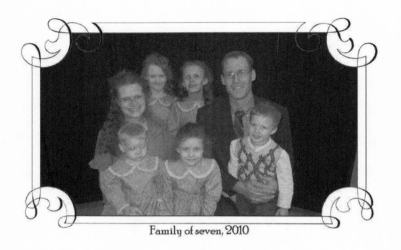

Family of seven, 2010

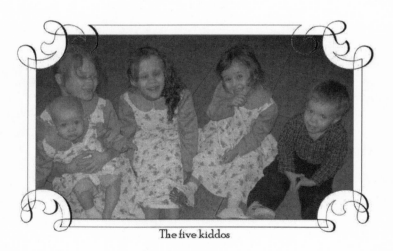

The five kiddos

Chapter Twelve

All Things Work Together for Good

All continued perfectly until I hit thirty-two weeks. The kids were playing tag, and as I walked across the room, one of them was running towards me, with her head down. She didn't see me and rammed right into my tummy with her head.

Instantly, I felt my uterus clinch up. I doubled over in pain and the contractions started. I got to the couch and curled up. I drank a quart of water and took some tinctures. Once Nathan got home, he prepared an Epsom salt bath for me.

From that point on, I had steady contractions. I was so close. I had wanted to make it the entire pregnancy without bed rest, but I had to go down. I spent the next four weeks on bed rest.

Several friends from church jumped in and helped me pick up the slack in the house. They also helped provide meals. Bed rest felt like a crushing blow because, at this point, I had expected to make it to the end of the pregnancy without it.

I came to the conclusion that the health changes I had made allowed my body to be strong enough to prevent preterm labor. But it wasn't quite enough to stop it once it was caused by trauma.

"I can't wait till I reach thirty-six weeks," I told Nathan. "I am looking forward to getting up. I wonder what Pam is going to say at our appointment next week."

Pam confirmed that the contractions had made some changes, preparing my body for labor. "It is hard to say what is going to happen. There are enough changes that you could go into labor and have the baby anytime now, but not so much that that is a sure thing. You could still go full term."

Little did I know that soon, I would be wishing I had gone full term!

That next month came and went. A few days before my due date arrived, the intensity of the contractions picked up. I started having extreme pelvic pressure. I knew labor was coming.

Within a few hours, contraction had increased to two to three minutes apart. Nathan stayed home from work and we called the midwife. We knew this was it! Or at least we THOUGHT we knew.

Labor continued. It was full blown, I was struggling to breathe through these contractions, but I never quite hit transition. The hours went by and as night approached, I was hopeful. So many people labored all day and then had their babies in the early morning. I expected the same for me.

I, however, labored all through the night. Morning came and still no baby. Labor dragged on. I was five centimeters dilated, so it had to be soon. Or did it?

Finally, labor just stopped. I was exhausted. I went to bed, expecting to wake up in transition. But I woke up to nothing.

During that day of labor, all the ligaments in my pelvis loosened up to get ready for birth. Birth stalled out, but the ligaments didn't tighten back.

From that point until birth, my tail bone kept slipping out of place. It would slip unexpectedly, and my legs would lock up. I couldn't move until Nathan would use his fist and manipulate the bone back into place.

I was counting on Lisa to be at my birth again, and a week later I sent her a message.

"Hi Lisa,

I am officially four, almost five days overdue, and I am feeling VERY, VERY done! Days are rough and I just don't have much energy left. My feet have been swelling a lot more the past few days.

I have had many more contractions since we last talked. Yesterday they picked way up and then in the night I was up for hours with tons of contractions that were really picking up in intensity. I also spent a lot of the day in the bathroom cleaning out. I was pretty sure that I wouldn't make it through the night. ... And then it stopped about 2 a.m. And today? Nothing! Seriously, not a single contraction more than just Braxton Hicks. Actually, this is the calmest my uterus has been in several weeks. Go figure...

So, I really have no idea what to expect. My mind tells me that it really can't be that much longer. But I am having a hard time convincing myself. ...

Hopefully, I will be calling soon!"

But it wasn't soon enough for me. Every step was excruciating. Bodies weren't made to walk around so dilated with the ligaments so loosened. I felt like my body was literally going to fall apart. Contractions came and went, but no labor.

Finally, two weeks after my labor experience and ten days past my due date, we decided that we couldn't keep this up. It was time to intervene.

Pam is usually slow to encourage doing things to initiate labor, but because of the situation, she was on board. I woke up that morning feeling great--for the first time in a very long time. We headed to see Pam and to get my membranes stripped.

"There is really not much for me to do," Pam told me. "I tried to strip them, but your body has already done most of it. You are ready to have this baby!"

Next we headed out to an herb shop to buy a tincture designed to help keep labor going. I started taking the tincture right away, and continued it every hour. We went to Costco and stocked up on some groceries and browsed the store. As I walked up and down the aisles, I had a few contractions here and there, but not much happened.

We made it home for lunch and I puttered around cleaning up the kitchen. I couldn't believe that even after stripping my membranes and taking multiple doses of the tincture, nothing was happening. "It's time for the next step!" I decided.

Castor oil! I had said I would never take it again, but I was desperate. I peeled several oranges and blended them with the oil. I was surprised at just how well the orange masked the oil. I got it down without bringing it back up.

About 6:00 p.m. the contractions picked up, and quickly were coming four to five minutes apart. About 9:00, Pam arrived and an hour later, my friends, Lisa and Christina, arrived as well. Once the ladies arrived, my contractions petered out. When I went in the other room, I would have a big contraction, but when I was being watched, there was next to nothing.

Pam said it looked like it wasn't happening yet, so she sent Lisa and Christina home and sent me to bed. Pam debated whether she should go on home but decided to sleep on the couch just in case.

I was asleep instantly, but woke an hour later with one strong contraction. I was only awake a couple minutes, before I was out again. I slept another hour and woke back up to head to the bathroom.

"Wow, that contraction felt like it really did something," I thought. I went back to bed and several minutes passed without anything. I felt another one and then I felt the familiar "pop" and a gush of water.

"Wake up now! The baby is coming!" I shook Nathan urgently. He jumped up and started to fill the tub. Pam heard the confusion and picked up her phone to call Lisa.

Another contraction hit and I panicked. I was afraid that I wouldn't be able to make it through this labor. How could I handle hours of this?

"I can't do this," I cried out. Pam dropped the phone and came running.

I rolled off the bed, got on my knees, laid my head on the bed, and started crying. The next contraction came, and I realized I needed to push. Amidst a flurry of confusion, my baby came in a single push.

Fourteen minutes and four contractions from the moment I first awoke, Pam was placing the baby in my arms. I held her close, basking in the love a mother feels for her new baby.

Pam helped me sit back, so that I could rest against the wall, and I realized that I didn't even know if it was a boy or girl! I held the baby up.

"It's a girl!" I laughed. "It's another girl. Her name is Ruth Abigail."

Nathan helped me up to the bed and I realized that the birth tub was about full.

"Should I get in the tub, now?" I joked. "I could go swimming."

As miserable as my labor and the time leading up to labor had been, I couldn't have asked for a more awesome birth! I expected that the postpartum would go just as smoothly, but I was wrong.

Ruthie latched on well and nursed like a pro. It seemed like we were going to have a great nursing experience, but within a day, I knew something was wrong. The nursing pain increased, and as time went by, I became bloody, raw, and cracked.

Eventually, Ruthie started to get agitated. I would cry in pain when she latched on, and then she would get frustrated and pull off, only to latch on and pull off again. I had shooting pains every time she tried to latch back on.

By the third day, we decided to go back in to see Pam, and she found the problem! Ruthie was tongue tied. Pam was able to clip the tie and we hoped that was the end of the trouble, but it wasn't.

As Ruthie would try to latch on, she would pull off and cry in frustration. I was so raw and open that I developed yeast and Ruthie got thrush.

The pain for both of us was so great that something had to change.

"I think it is time to pull out the pump," I lamented. I pumped enough milk for Ruthie and carefully fed her with a little cup. It was slow and tedious, but once she was satisfied, she settled down and slept. Thus began the cycle of trying to nurse, pump, feed, etc.

"Feeding Ruthie is a full time job," I complained to Nathan. "I am just so exhausted I can't even think anymore. I am supposed to be staying off my feet??? Ha, that's a joke. And I am so done with the pain. I just want to be done." But I was far from being done.

My house was falling apart around me. The church was delivering meals for supper, which was a blessing. I don't think we would have eaten much otherwise.

Gradually Ruthie's thrush cleared up, but I was healing much slower. I kept exacerbating the problem each time I fed her or pumped. As Ruthie healed, we tried to transition to more nursing and less pumping. As my body tried to adjust to the transfer away from the pump, it hit a snag: mastitis.

"I think I am going to die," I moaned to Nathan, as I tossed and turned, alternating from burning up to freezing cold. It took two days for the mastitis to run its course, but eventually the infection worked its way out. I used castor oil packs on my breast to help fight the infection.

Once the mastitis was over, life got smoother--for a little while. Ruthie figured out how to nurse well, and the pain cleared up. By now Ruthie was two weeks old and I didn't even bother to try to stay down anymore. There was way too much to do to bother. I figured that I had already been up so much, it wouldn't make a difference now.

I jumped back into life. Everyone was happy to have a new baby. She kept everyone smiling and happy. I pulled out new school curriculum and we started setting up schedules and plans. Unfortunately, my schedule didn't last very long.

"Something is wrong," I fretted. "I don't know what it is, but something just isn't right. I feel like I am about to fall out."

I called Pam again and we eventually figured out what was wrong. I had a prolapse. This was not just any prolapse--this was a triple prolapse--vaginal, rectal and cervical prolapse at once. No wonder I felt like everything was about to fall out. It was.

Pam told me that the conventional treatment was surgery, but that didn't come without some risks. She encouraged me to call Lisa about some more natural options.

Lisa encouraged me to purchase a Kegalmaster, an exercise device designed to take Kegals to a whole new level. Another friend recommended a Pilates Pelvic Floor workout. I put the two together and came up with a plan.

I worked hard at doing the things that would help my prolapse. Little by little, I could feel things moving back into place. For a while it was pretty painful to be on my feet, but as I did the various exercises, the pain subsided. Eventually, I reversed the problem all together!

It was such a relief to finally be back on my feet. I jumped back into the school, schedule and plans that I had started. I was ready for a new season of life!

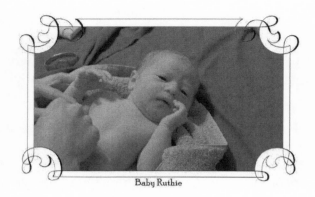

Baby Ruthie

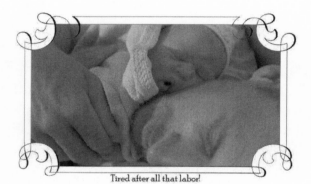

Tired after all that labor!

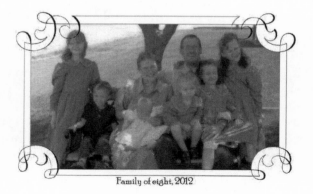

Family of eight, 2012

Chapter Thirteen

Grace in My Weakness

"Are you ready to load the van?" Nathan asked me.

"Getting closer," I replied, as I glanced over the kitchen and grabbed a few more items I thought we might need.

Nathan loaded the van while I got the kids up and ready to leave. I had breakfast ready to eat in the van, and food for the next couple of days on the road. We headed out towards Colorado to help Nathan's family with the wheat harvest.

I was happy when we arrived and was looking forward to a good night's sleep.

"Man, I am sore," I stretched, trying to get the knots out of my muscles. "These must not be very good beds."

Over the next few days I woke up sorer and sorer. Nathan was working hard in the fields, and I was just taking care of the kids. He was the one who should be sore, not me!

Every morning I fed the kids, then loaded them up, and took them over to Nathan's parents' house. I stayed there until time to head back for the night.

"I really should go now," I told Nathan's mom. But I just didn't feel like getting up. It seemed like a big task to get everybody out the door to where we were staying a quarter mile away. Each evening, I found myself procrastinating more and more.

I didn't think too much about it at the time. I figured that the trip had taken a toll on me and I knew that my body had gone through a lot. I figured I would just push through it and move on.

But I didn't. I couldn't.

We were in Colorado for two weeks, and the pain and exhaustion continued. I was able to function well enough and I was looking forward to getting home and settled. I assumed I would feel better once I got back into normal life. But after we got home, I realized that was just the beginning!

A few weeks later I posted on my blog:

"The last few weeks have been very challenging for me, and by default, my whole family. I began to have some serious health symptoms in early August. I began to be in pain over my whole body. It has been pain 24/7. Also with the pain came extreme weakness, dizziness and a myriad of other symptoms. Some days, the severity of it has been debilitating. Some days, the pain is all over. Some days it settles in my joints, so I am unable to straighten my legs, arm or fingers. As we look at the various symptoms, it

appears that we may be dealing with some sort of autoimmune disorder.

I have an appointment this Friday for a full body evaluation. They specialize in the reversal of chronic illness. We were happy to find this center, as they are MDs, who can provide any conventional care and treatment we may need. However, they also focus on treating naturally and getting to the root of the problems, rather than just treating symptoms. It was an answer to prayer to find both of those with one caregiver.

I would appreciate your prayers for my family and me, as we try to find some answer to what is wrong with me and we begin the journey to healing."

Soon I had an update:

"We saw the doctor on Friday. She did lots of tests and got some preliminary answers. She is a very interesting doctor, and I think that she will be able to lead me on the path to regaining my heath well.

First off, I do have fibromyalgia and chronic fatigue syndrome. I also have toxin overload. The cells in my body are not working correctly. They are unable to eliminate toxins as they should, plus they are not able to adequately receive the nutrients that come in.

The toxic overload and cell issues can lead to many, many problems, including other auto-immune disorders, as I suspected. We will be doing more tests and stuff to get some more answers as to what those things are in my case."

Soon, our life revolved around appointments, tests, needles and pain. But I wasn't getting better.

Within a month, we had some more answers:

"We had a good appointment last Friday, and we got a lot of information. Let's start with the Mitochondrial Dysfunction. The Mitochondria is the part of your cells that produces energy. I have a significant amount of Oxidative Stress and my Mitochondria are damaged. The cell walls are breaking down and they are unable to deal with the toxins that come in. And, by default, they are unable to produce the energy that my body needs to function.

Other test results are showing that my intestinal tract is working on a high level of stress, even when not under stress. Basically, it is allowing the toxins that go in my body, and would normally be eliminated, to seep back into my body. This level of toxic overload is causing the oxidative stress and the damage to the Mitochondria.

So, it is working like a vicious cycle. The more the toxins are seeping in, the more my cells are damaged. The more cellular damage, the less they can handle the toxins. Thus, I have a very high level of oxidative stress. Also, because of all this damage, my body is unable to assimilate the nutrients that I do take in, which is hindering the cells from recovering.

All of this causes levels of inflammation in my body, and that is the cause of the high levels of pain. My joints are especially targeted. This is also why I am so extremely fatigued and exhausted.

I told Nathan that it feels like I have a vice grip on my joints. Some days it is so tight I can't stand it. Some days it loosens up for a bit of relief. But it is still there.

So, all in all, I am very sick, in pain, and can barely function. Basically my body reached a point that it could not handle the internal damage, and it crashed."

All of this information was just pieces of the puzzle. We were still looking for the cause. In spite of all the tests and treatments, I was getting worse. Soon, I considered myself an invalid. I struggled to take a step even with the help of a walker.

Months passed. The neurological symptoms got worse and I struggled to form sentences and to even interact with people. My brain was slow to process any information, and I began to slur my words.

This was a scary time. I thought that I was dying. I figured, at the rate I was going down, I had two to three months to live. I had previously gone through so much pain and challenges, but nothing compared to this. The pain was so unbearable that I came to the point that death felt like a welcome relief.

Nathan knelt on the floor in front of me. It took all my effort to raise my hand and pat him on the head. "It will be OK," I said, "You will make it. God is in control."

This time I didn't say "we." I didn't think I would make it.

Nathan put his head down on my chest and wept. I stroked his head a couple times before the weakness overtook me and my hand dropped. I had no energy left to do anything but lie there.

177

My heart surged with gratefulness that I was married to Nathan. I knew that my kids would be well taken care of.

But once again, God had other plans for me! The newest test gave us the results that answered so many questions: Lyme Disease.

We were able to pinpoint a time, about twelve years earlier, when I was traveling through Tennessee and I walked through a field and was bitten by nearly twenty ticks. Most of the ticks were removed immediately after the walk, but a couple of them slipped by my search and I didn't discover them until several days had passed.

This was a prime setup to contract Lyme and the many years of being undiagnosed would explain the severity of the current symptoms. Lyme is known for hiding and silently causing damage.

Now that we knew what we were dealing with, we were better armed to treat me. God directed us to a clinic in Kansas. The Hansa Center treats chronic illness and specializes in Lyme Disease. We researched their philosophy of treatment and decided to give it a try.

About this time I conceived, but God chose to take this child quickly. We grieved the life of this little one quietly, only sharing with people close to us. I didn't want guilt placed on me by people who would have thought that I shouldn't have gotten pregnant.

The Hansa Center has a two-week program on site and, during that program, they help their patients set up an at-home protocol. Our whole family headed up to Kansas.

God worked out every detail of this trip. He paved the way financially, and He used this trip to bring lifelong friends into our life. And God used this trip to initiate my healing.

At the end of the first week, I was able to put my cane down and walk! By the end of the second week, I made muffins in the kitchen. I can't begin to express how wonderful it felt to be given back the gift of functioning. I could do nothing before I went and now I could function somewhat.

I came home with a new lease on life! I wasn't completely healed, but I had set the stage for healing to occur. I like to compare it to a badly broken bone. Until you go to the doctor and get that bone set, the problem will get worse, and recovery just isn't going to happen. Once you have that bone set, now it is ready to heal.

The goal of the Hansa Center was to put my body into the position to be able to heal. Once I was home, I began a whole new season of life. My life was taken over by therapies, treatments, supplements, etc. It was challenging to balance what I could do and what I needed to do, with all the time-consuming treatments that were needed

I did have some days that I had to stay completely down, but on my good days, I could get up and cook some meals. I was able to take care of the children, but I was not able to do almost any household chores.

When I would do chores, the Lyme symptoms would flare, the pain would increase, and I would go back down for days. Over the next year, I felt like I was walking a fine line. I wanted to improve and strengthen my body. I wanted to be able to do more. But if I did too much, I would have a setback. Every day I worked at figuring out just how much I could do without doing too much.

Most days I was so grateful for the improvements! I praised God for the reduction of pain to a tolerable level. I praised Him for the ability to walk and do a few things.

But other days were harder. I still struggled with my limitations. I was very weak, and there was so much I couldn't do. I had to learn to either depend on others to help me, or to be content with things undone. Both were hard.

One of my goals during this time was to work on keeping my children's heart. Daily I fought the temptation to wallow in self-pity. I tried to choose to be joyful, to love my children, to be a good mom. I wanted them to look back at this time without regrets.

A year later, I went back to Hansa for the second two-week program. My doctor was happy to see how many of the improvements had held over the past year.

I saw significant improvement. I went from being able to function at a minimal level to being able to work diligently, on occasion, and function at a higher level.

My pain levels were reduced even more and my neurological challenges really saw the improvement! After that visit in February, 2014, my recovery was taken to a whole new level!

I still had to keep up with my treatments at home, but I could live life around them. And I was so grateful.

But I am getting ahead of my story!

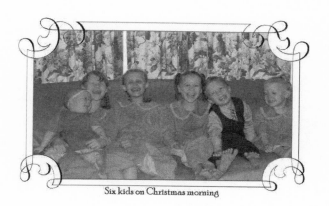

Six kids on Christmas morning

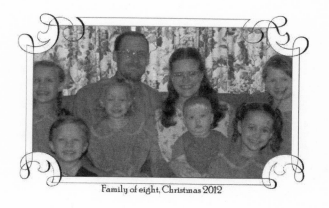

Family of eight, Christmas 2012

Chapter Fourteen

It Will be Worth it All

Shortly after I returned from my first visit to the Hansa Center, I had to have jaw surgery. The root canals I had done previously were infected into the bone. The dentist needed to remove the teeth and scrape out the infection from the bone.

The recovery was painful, and even though it had been several years since I had taken any conventional medication, I took the prescription pain killers.

A week later, we got the news! I was pregnant! I was surprised that I conceived so soon after the last miscarriage. We were excited to celebrate a new life as we entered this new stage of life--recovery from the Lyme Disease. But I also fretted about all the medications I had taken during and after my surgery, while I was pregnant and didn't know it yet.

In all my research, I found some connections from the Lyme to my pregnancy issues. I wondered if the many miscarriages and the preterm labor were directly related to the Lyme Disease.

"It is not the Lyme caused those things, per se," I explained to a friend. "But I do think that the damage caused to my body from the Lyme did cause them. I am excited to see how the Lyme treatment will affect this pregnancy."

I had high hopes for a better pregnancy and no preterm labor. My hopes were tested when I started spotting, but that was short lived. The bleeding stopped and I took another pregnancy test--still two lines. Over the next few days, I took several more tests--all positive.

I spent a week or so taking it easy, but the bleeding never returned. All was well! We rejoiced that our baby had survived that scare, and we were ready to see how this pregnancy would play out.

One of the obvious benefits was that the morning sickness did not hit as usual. There was nothing for at least six weeks and, after that, just occasional twinges. It was all tolerable, and I was amazed at how much a change in diet affected morning sickness!

Pretty soon, people were asking us if we were going to find out whether we were going to have a boy or a girl. My first inclination was to say no. We had decided against doing a sonogram last time, and why should we go back on that decision?

But, I continued to fret about whether everything was going to be ok. I had done so much in those first weeks of pregnancy that I would have never done, had I known I was pregnant. I worried that I had harmed our baby.

As I thought through the decision of the sonogram, I remembered that we had decided that as long there
184

wasn't any risk to not doing it, we wouldn't, and that we would only consider it if there was a reason we needed to confirm or deny a problem.

I realized that all my fretting about whether my baby would be OK was really bothering me. I just couldn't get past thinking about that. I couldn't imagine having that level of fretting through the entire pregnancy.

"Nathan, I've decided!" I announced one day.

"Oh, really?" Nathan asked with a chuckle.

"Yes, I've made an executive decision." Then I added, "If you approve, of course."

"Oh, and what might that be?" he wondered.

"I've decided that the detriment of not knowing if all my decisions hurt our baby is worse than the risks of harm from a sonogram. I have decided that I want to go ahead and do it. I need to know that everything is ok."

"Well then, go ahead and call and make an appointment."

So I did! We found a mobile sonogram guy that several friends had used and he came right to our home! I waited anxiously, as he set up his equipment. I felt a little sick with dread as to what we would find.

He placed the wand on my tummy and instantly we could see our baby dancing around. That was one sight that never ceased to amaze me!

He checked out a few details and told me that the baby looked perfect. A weight lifted from my heart. I was so relieved!

Then he announced the news that everyone was waiting for: another BOY! Andy especially was thrilled to not be the only boy in the sea of girls.

"I wished it could have been quintuplet boys, so we could be the same as the girls," Andy said, "but I guess I will be happy with just one boy."

You would think that with just one boy and five girls, we would find boy names easier. But this time I had a girl's name chosen and we weren't any closer to deciding on a boy's name. We discussed names around the dinner table.

"How about Fred?"

"Let's name him Harry."

"I still like Boanerges."

The talk went on and on, but we weren't getting anywhere.

"Alright, already, let's be serious," I exclaimed. "I want to get this child named now!"

We eventually settled on a name: Philip Tyndale Marr.

I was thrilled to finally have a name and to know who my son was.

One day, one of my kids said, "Momma, I dreamed that your baby popped out and then your tummy was not so fat!" I wished it were that easy--on both accounts!

On September 28, I updated my Facebook:

"I will be 34 weeks along on Tuesday. We just realized that this is the first time EVER that I have reached this point in pregnancy and have still been on my feet. I've been on bed rest with all the others. Praise God for His mercy and for not having premature labor!

I do still struggle with my Lyme Disease daily, BUT my improvement over last year is very significant. I believe that the Lyme was the cause of many of my pregnancy problems, and I am excited to see the improvement this time, now that I am treating the Lyme."

A friend of ours, Rebekah, came to stay with us on and off for several months. We enjoyed having her company, and it was helpful to have her help around the house and with the children.

The time for Philip to be born was quickly approaching. My babies seem to have a habit of trying to come long before they actually come. I was concerned about how to keep labor on track once it started.

On November 6 I wrote, *"I can tell Philip is getting bigger! He doesn't have enough room for all his acrobatic feats anymore. Now he just squirms, and we can all see my tummy flip flop. He seems ready to come, if contractions tell me anything. We just have to get them from being just enough to keep me awake at night to actually getting him out!"*

I decided that this time I was not going to just stand by and endure the start and stop labor. If labor started, I was going to help it finish.

Sure enough, as my due date approached, contractions picked up. I was getting a little antsy to get all the work I wanted done before the baby was here--especially getting my bathroom and bedroom scrubbed!

I was counting on Nathan to help me on his day off, but then he announced that he had plans. Cautiously, I asked him what they were. I was afraid something had come up and he wouldn't be home, after all.

Nathan grinned and replied, "Clean our bedroom, scrub our bathroom, fill a birth pool, put you in it, get Philip out, and go to bed."

"I like your kind of thinking!" I laughed back. But it wasn't quite time for the getting Philip out part.

A midwife appointment estimated Philip to be over seven pounds, and I was dilated to three. He was going to be one of my bigger babies, and he would be coming soon!

Whenever my due date is coming up and I ask Nathan when he thinks the baby will be born, he always throws out a random date in the far distant future, and I usually end up throwing a pillow at him. But on November 7, his tone changed.

"Do you think that Philip will be born tomorrow?" I asked into the phone.

"Yes," Nathan replied.

"What did you just say?" I said in surprise

"That he will be born tomorrow," Nathan repeated.

"And how are we going to make sure that happens?" I wondered.

"We will put you on the trampoline and make you jump till he comes out."

Nathan laughed, but he was too far away for me to throw a pillow.

Contractions continued on and off for the next few days, and I decided that it was time to keep things going. With all my past preterm labor and so much effort to stop labor over and over, I felt like I had trained my body to stop labor before it was done. My body didn't seem to be able to stop that cycle.

On the morning of November 10, I decided to go ahead with the castor oil. Nathan took all of the kids to church, and our friend, Rebekah, stayed with me.

I made a chocolate peanut butter smoothie to mask the flavor of the castor oil, but I put in too many ingredients and ended up with two full glasses to drink. I took the glasses, a straw, a good book, and lay on my bed.

It took me over an hour to get the smoothies down, and by the time I was done, I never wanted to look at a chocolate peanut butter smoothie again! Once it was down, I took a nap.

When I woke up, I was cramping, but there was no sign of real labor contractions. I felt pretty sick and yucky, so I stayed in bed. I also took my tincture to help keep labor going. I wanted to rest as much as possible to be ready for labor, but by evening, I got up and puttered around the house.

I was cramping a lot, and had some strong contractions, but the whole day went by with no baby. Things were picking up late in the evening, and we called Pam and Lisa to give them the heads up.

I went to bed about 10:00. I had already figured out that my body had a pattern of trying to go into labor, going to sleep, and then waking up in full labor. This time, I only got one hour of sleep.

I woke up to a contraction and I knew this was it! I had asked Nathan to fill the birth pool for me, just in case, but I was not interested in it now. Since I was now doing daily detox baths, and they were so miserable, I just couldn't equate being in the water with comfort.

I just wanted my birth ball in front of my bed, so that I could rest my head while I rocked my hips. Nathan called Lisa and Pam and told them that it was time.

Before I went to bed I had set up a crock pot on warm, filled with water and Young Living Lavender Oil. With each contraction, Nathan grabbed a new rag, squeezed it out and held it over my tummy. I made sure he used two hands so that the rag could touch as much surface as possible.

It was amazing just how much the lavender oil and heat combination soothed the pain and helped me relax! It would take me from feeling like I was about to panic to feeling, "I can do this!"

An hour and a half went by and the contractions remained consistent. I knew the end was near. Pretty soon Pam gave me the go ahead to push, and push I did. But nothing happened. I pushed again during the next contraction and then again.

Pretty soon, I felt like my control was slipping. I realized that something wasn't quite right. I started to panic and felt like I couldn't handle it.

"He's stuck," I cried. Pam checked me and I was right. He was indeed stuck. There was a lip of cervix that was holding him back. Pam decided to hold it back while I pushed.

The pain was excruciating but short lived. Within minutes I was holding Philip!

Once again I experienced the awe that washes over a new mother with her baby. That surge of love that is so amazing that words can't describe it!

Philip was given an Apgar score of 10/10. To top off a no bed rest pregnancy with that kind of a score felt like an amazing feat. Nathan helped me back on the bed and I took Philip to nurse him.

"He won't latch on," I fretted to Nathan. This time we weren't going to wait and hope it worked itself out. We handed him over to Pam, who confirmed that he was tongue tied. Pam clipped the tie quickly. It was a relief to know we had caught it and that I wouldn't have to suffer like last time.

Philip didn't cooperate at first. He wouldn't latch on; he just wanted to snuggle and sleep. I kept trying and trying, with my stress level high, but eventually he figured it out. Less than twenty-four hours after his birth,

Philip was a champion nurser! We never had another problem with his eating.

Philip was the happiest, most contented baby I had ever seen. A few days after birth, the whole family came down with the flu. I tried to keep the other children away as much as possible, while I took natural remedies and essential oils to keep the germs away. For a week, I was able to keep Philip and me from getting sick, but eventually it caught up with us.

Philip and I both got a light case, but the flu with a newborn is concerning, no matter how light. I could hear the congestion start to build up in his lungs. I used Young Living RC essential oil (which stands for Respiratory Congestion) on his chest. I saw immediate results. His little chest opened up and he could breathe more easily.

Any time Philip's breathing started to sound concerning, I gave him another rub of RC oil. We praise God that the oils worked so well. He sailed through the sickness without any cause for worry. He stayed happy and content through the whole thing. What a relief!

Once we made it through the postpartum time and had all the sickness behind us, I tried to get back into the swing of life. Rebekah went back to her home and I was on my own.

I quickly realized that I did not have the ability to do all I needed to do. In spite of daily therapy, my body was still struggling with the Lyme disease. I posted an update on Facebook, so my friends would know what had been going on.

"This month will be one year since I was diagnosed with Chronic Lyme Disease. What a journey it has been! It is ironic how such a devastating diagnosis could be such a relief, but it was.

A year ago, I was pretty much an invalid. I struggled to lift my feet up for a step. Walking was slow and tortuous, and that was with the help of a walker. I was in chronic pain 24/7--pain so bad that at times I would beg God to let me die. My neurological symptoms would sometimes be so bad that I struggled to carry on a conversation and I would slur my words. I felt like I was losing my ability to speak AND to think, and to function in any way. And thus was my life for 6 months.

I did not tell anyone this, but I went down so fast that I truly believed I only had a few months to live. No one besides Nathan really had any idea how bad I was physically. Even those who lived closest to me only saw me at my very best.

And then I was diagnosed with Chronic Lyme Disease, and that is where my uphill journey started. Some might think that after a year of treatment, I should not be struggling as much as I do. But I know the truth. I know that I have come so very far in this year that I couldn't ask for more significant improvement in that time frame. I do pray that this next year brings even more healing and recovering, but in the meantime, my ability to live life has been restored.

Healing from Chronic Lyme is a very slow process. It has been compared to a house with termites. Once the termites are dead, there is still significant damage to the foundation of the house. The Lyme spirochete burrows into all the

193

parts of the body, and even after they are all dead, there is still much damage done to the body. It is a slow process to restore it.

My journey started at the Hansa Center, a clinic dealing with Chronic Illness, where I went through their two-week program. I arrived in the condition I explained above, and two weeks later I WALKED out. I estimate that in those two weeks, they reduced my symptoms by 75%. If you could have seen the difference, you would realize just how miraculous it was.

That was the beginning of significant amounts of therapies and treatments at home. It felt as though my life revolved around doing stuff to help my body recover. And it did.

I expected to go home and make progress from there, but God had different and better plans for me. He knew that what we really needed was baby Philip. I continued to improve for a month, until I got pregnant. At that point, the recovery slowed and then eventually halted. I continued some of my treatments, and rather than help me recover, those treatments helped me to maintain where I was. If I skipped even a day, symptoms would start to return--I would begin to stumble, slur words, pain would increase, etc.

"Even with any setback I had during the pregnancy, I am still vastly better than I was last year. We feel like all of the effort that my body was previously putting into recovering, was now being put into making a baby, and that my treatments were only helping me to hold onto what I had already gained. I believe that from here on out, we will begin to see more and more healing over this next year. I am hoping to return back to the Hansa Center within a few

months to jump start the healing again, though I don't know if that will be possible. Meanwhile, I will continue to do what I can here at home to continue healing.

I sit here with Philip (now 3 weeks) in my arms, and I thank God for the many blessings that He has poured on us this year. In some ways, it seems like we have had so many struggles and trials, but God has been so faithful to us in the midst of it, and we praise Him."

The next couple of months I struggled to get up and going, but my physical limitations held me back. We decided that I needed to go back to Hansa sooner rather than later. We scheduled an appointment for February, 2014.

Dr. Jowdy told me that the first time I had visited, I was like a car that didn't run. This time I was like a running car with just enough gas to get around the corner.

That analogy fit perfectly with how I felt. Our goal was to get my body gassed up and give it enough energy to function again.

The two-week program was just as successful as the first time! I left the Hansa Center feeling like a new person. I still had some limitations, and I still had to do my treatments every day, but I now had enough energy to function.

I came home with a new lease on life. I started a new school year with the children. I worked on getting my house organized and back in order. It was thrilling to be able to do even the most basic chores. One thing I've learned in life was that we don't know how much we value something till it is taken from us.

LESSONS LEARNED

I look back over my life before I got married. I remember a friend congratulating me on my engagement, but also lamenting the struggles I would have to go through. I didn't understand at the time. I could see no struggles connected with marriage to Nathan.

Eventually, I learned. No, my struggle was not my marriage. But with my marriage, I opened the door for a new set of life circumstances and a whole new level of challenges that I would never have faced being single.

But that wasn't the only thing I learned. I learned to trust in God. I learned what God meant when He said that He would work all things out for our good. I learned that even though man plans his way, the Lord directs his steps.

I had so many dreams, plans and expectations, and God took us down an entirely different path. Then I assumed that the trials that came our way would end our ability to have the children our original dreams contained.

But God knew better. I was reminded again that man's wisdom is foolishness to God and that often our reasoning goes against God's perfect plan.

I look back over my twelve years of marriage and I thank God. I thank God for His mercy on us. I thank Him for His grace during the trials, for the lessons He taught us. I thank God for overriding our logic and pouring out His blessings on us. I thank Him for the children He has given us. I thank Him for life!

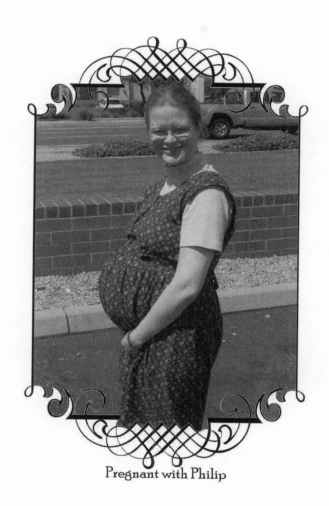

Pregnant with Philip

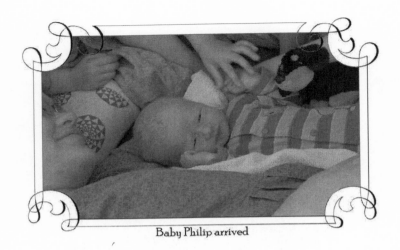

Baby Philip arrived

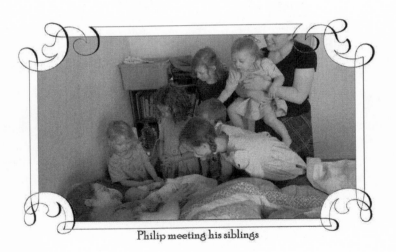

Philip meeting his siblings

Chapter Fifteen

Preterm Labor Guide and Other Pregnancy Tips

Imagine we are sitting across the table chatting and sipping herbal tea together. If you were to ask me what you should do to help prevent or treat preterm labor, these are the things I would tell you.

EPSOM SALT We've all heard of people going to the hospital and getting magnesium sulfate via IV to stop preterm labor. Do you know what Epsom Salt is? Magnesium sulfate! It is so much more comfortable to absorb all that good stuff through the skin, rather than through an IV. Then you don't have to have all those nasty side effects!

Add 2+ cups Epsom Salt to a warm bath. A couple of drops of lavender oil are a great addition. Relax and soak. A half hour would be the minimum you would want to soak to start getting the benefits, but one to one and a half hours would be better. This is a great way to keep your uterus relaxed and prevent preterm labor. It can even halt preterm labor in the early stages. I recommend this daily if you are at high risk.

If for any reason baths don't work for you, Epsom salt foot baths are a great alternative. For prevention or minor contractions, I set a container on the floor and sat on the couch. However, there were times I also needed to stay lying down. My husband would set up a chair beside my bed with the water bath. I would lie on the bed, near the edge and have my knees up, and my feet in the container. It wasn't the most comfortable position, but I did use it more than once to halt labor.

WATER Drink, drink, drink!!! Often, even slight dehydration can bring on contractions. Aim for a gallon of water a day. I like to fill four quarts of water in the evening and aim for one throughout the night and three the following day. Having the water ready the night before helps me prevent procrastination.

You can doctor up your water a bit to make sure that you are getting enough electrolytes and not just flushing out your system. A squeeze of lemon juice and a touch of honey is a great way to do that. There are powders that you can purchase and add to your water. You can also make a pregnancy tea. You can prepare a weak tea and then drink lots of it.

You want to be sure to focus on making your water intake mostly between meals. If you drink it all during meals, you will dilute your digestive enzymes and make it harder for your body to process your food.

PROTEIN Sometimes contractions are your body's cry for food. You should be proactive to get good protein in your system. I like to cook up meat to freeze in snack size portions. Every few days, I would take out a bunch of servings to defrost. I would eat it cold from the fridge. Cheese, hard boiled eggs, nuts, and peanut butter are all things easy to have on hand. Homemade granola bars can be made to have an extra boost of protein. I found that having a variety of things prepared ahead of time helped me to be proactive to get enough protein.

And when I say protein, I mean protein! When I eat eggs, I eat at least three! I try to eat a generous serving of protein with each meal, and I eat protein snacks scattered through the day. If you don't feel like you are eating too much protein, you are probably not eating enough!

Eating some carbs with your protein will help it stick, keep your body working well, and help reduce morning sickness. Some ideas would be a tuna sandwich, celery with nut butter, apple with cheese, granola and milk, beans with cheese, and smoothies. Purchased snacks, such as a Lara Bar are also helpful to keep on hand.

CALORIES Do not restrict calories. Calories are energy and you will need all the energy you can get! Excessive calories are not the problem. The problem lies in the quality of the calories. Make sure every calorie you eat is

201

benefiting your body. Don't pass up an avocado so you can justify a Snickers bar. One feeds you, the other tears you down. They are not equal. Make your focus be on making wise choices rather than the quantity of the calories.

You will want to try to get some calories every two hours. This will help to keep your body going without crashing. You can see the section above for some quick snack options. Be proactive and plan ahead, so that you always have something available when you need it.

If you haven't planned, you are likely to open the fridge, and close it right back and walk away, or make a bad choice and eat something that you shouldn't. It doesn't need to be a full meal every two hours, but eat something!

HERBAL TINCTURES There are a lot of different herbal tinctures that are good muscle relaxants. These made a huge difference for me! I like to have a variety and to mix-match what I have to multiply the benefits. Often, they do the same thing, but approach it with a different ingredient. Also, your body can adjust to an herb if taken too often and you won't get as much benefit. These can be used as needed.

When I was just having hints of contractions, using them two to three times a day was plenty. If contractions began to pick up, I would take one every fifteen to thirty minutes, rotating them to try to calm them down quickly. These are all the ones I use.

Singles:

Cramp Bark

Black Haw

False Unicorn

Blends:

Welcome Womb

Carry On Relief

Carry on

Cramp Relief

Crampbark, False Unicorn, Welcome Womb, and Carry On Relief are all available at www.inhishands.com and would be good ones to start with. Several of the blends have the single ingredients as one of the ingredients, so you would be getting those specific herbs.

Some of the herbs are alcohol tinctures and some are glycerin based. If you have a preference to one or the other, that is fine. I prefer to rotate between the two.

Be sure that you do *not* choose any tinctures designed for preventing cramping after birth (such as AfterEase). These tinctures contain ingredients to help expel whatever is left in the uterus and would be dangerous for pregnancy.

203

CALCIUM AND MAGNESIUM (and other minerals) These work together as a muscle relaxant. You often hear of athletes using a combination of these two to reduce muscle cramping. It works the same for labor contractions. I use these in fairly high doses. My favorite source of magnesium is Natural Calm. It is a powder that you mix into water and drink, and is very absorbable to your body. The minerals will help keep your electrolytes balanced and your body functioning correctly.

PROGESTERONE CREAM If you already know that you are at high risk for preterm labor, or if you have a hard time carrying your baby in early pregnancy, you should start using a natural progesterone cream as soon as you suspect pregnancy. I used a natural progesterone. The NOW brand was my favorite for the most cost efficient, yet clearly gave results. I have recently started using Young Living Progessence, which is a serum rather than a cream. I recommend either option.

Rub the progesterone over your lower abdomen twice a day. The raised progesterone levels can help your body maintain pregnancy. If your risk is mainly early miscarriage, continue using the progesterone till about fifteen weeks and then slowly wean yourself off. At that point, your placenta begins its own production of extra progesterone, and that is enough for most women.

If you are at risk for preterm labor, you should continue the progesterone until it is safe for your baby to be born. This could prevent the need for synthetic progesterone shots, and the higher level of progesterone triggers your body into knowing that it is not time for the baby to be born.

FAT High quality, healthy fats are essential. Some of these come in the form of supplements, and some are simply food.

Unrefined coconut oil should be a staple in your diet. It will keep you healthy, and it is amazingly beneficial to the development of your little one. Some people eat it off a spoon, but I could never stomach that. There are so many ways to include it in your diet. You can bake and cook with it, replacing it with whatever fat your recipe calls for. But you want to get some raw coconut oil in you.

One of the easiest ways for me to eat it is to make candy. Add peppermint oil and honey for peppermint patties. Add honey and peanut butter for fudge. Switch that up by adding cocoa powder for a yummy chocolate.

Cod liver oil should be your most essential supplement. I recommend Green Pastures Fermented Cod Liver Oil.

You should also be getting plenty of butter. Butter your toast, butter your vegetables. Be generous with your butter. Slather it on, knowing that you are benefiting your little one.

RED RASPBERRY LEAF TEA I like to make a blend of raspberry leaf tea, alfalfa, nettles, and peppermint leaf. This gives your body an infusion of bone-building minerals to help your little one develop. The raspberry leaf works as a uterine tonic preparing your uterus for labor, making it work more efficiently, and reducing contraction pain.

This is a little controversial during the main part of your pregnancy. Some say to avoid it if you are at risk for preterm labor, while others say it helps prevent preterm labor. I recommend that you do your own research and talk to your caregiver, so that you can make an informed decision. After thirty-six weeks, I highly recommend that everyone drink at least a quart of this liquid gold per day.

Personally, the controversy kept me from drinking it till thirty-six weeks in most of my pregnancies. However, after I researched it with my last baby, I drank it throughout the entire pregnancy.

DON'T HOLD IT When you need to use the bathroom ... go! Don't hold it. Sometimes, when you are fighting contractions, it feels counterproductive to drink lots of water and keep getting up to go to the bathroom. It is tempting to either lay low on the water intake or hold it as long as you can. Both are counterproductive and will cause much more harm than getting up will do.

When your bladder is full, it puts pressure on the uterus and triggers contractions. It can also increase the risk of bladder infections.

INFECTIONS Infections can cause preterm labor. If you are having early contractions, evaluate yourself for possible infections. Gum and bladder infections are often causes of preterm labor. Treat those and work hard on keeping your immune system strong, so that your body can fight off any unknown infections or prevent new ones.

PROBIOTICS Making sure you get enough probiotics will make your body happy. They will help your body properly deal with the food you eat and get the most benefit from it. They will also help your body eliminate it. Getting those toxins moved out will make a big difference in how you feel over all.

Studies have also shown that taking probiotics will significantly reduce your risk of Group B Strep

HEMORRHOID CARE I used to use witch hazel on small cotton pads and make my own "tucks." They worked well, but I found that I like using Young Living essential oils even better. I used a salve base and googled which oils helped with hemorrhoids. I chose among the ones I already owned and added them into the salve. I used this several times a day and it was extremely soothing.

EXERCISE Walk, walk, walk unless you are on bed rest with preterm labor. But bed rest or not, exercise is essential to the well-being of your body. I read once that one month on complete bed rest can age your body seven years. You don't want that!

If you are having a healthy pregnancy, you can likely continue doing what you always do. If you are at risk for preterm labor, you will have to be proactive in using your muscles and preventing atrophy. You can hold your arms up and do butterflies, do ankle twists. Just make a special effort to do whatever movement that you can do without triggering contractions. Sure, you will be limited, but better to keep doing the few things you can do than to lose the muscle that you could keep. It may feel wearying, but in the end, you will not regret it!

STAY DOWN My biggest advice for after birth is to stay down. I can't state enough how essential this is to the healing of your body! First, your cervix has dilated ten centimeters, and all of your internal organs are sitting on and placing pressure on the cervix. It takes six weeks for that to close up.

Also, when the placenta separates from your uterus, it leaves a dinner plate sized open wound. If that wound was on the outside of our body, we would protect it and treat it carefully. Since it is on the inside, we can easily forget it and pretend like it is no big deal.

Many ladies see an increase in bleeding at two to three weeks, when they start having more activity. Often, that bleeding is caused by the wound being broken open--as if the scab was picked off. We need to be very careful to protect our body from any unnecessary straining or pressure as that heals.

Ideally, I believe that a woman should stay completely down for two full weeks. I try to spend the first week in my bedroom and only get up for the bathroom. The second week, I will come out on the couch to interact with the family more, but will retreat to the bedroom as needed.

Weeks three and four, I start getting up cautiously in small amounts. I will eat at the table and sit up on the couch, change toddler diapers, etc., but I still stay down as much as possible. Weeks five and six are the transition into regular activity. By the end of week six, you should be ready for jumping into life again.

I believe that this level of care is necessary to take care of and protect our bodies and will help prevent damage that will jeopardize our future children.

AFTER BIRTH CARE After Ease--I love this tincture! After Ease helps reduce the afterbirth pains. I was able to eliminate pain medicine and replace it with After Ease. It is safe enough to take as often as you want.

Corn bags are great for after-birth cramps. You can heat them up in a microwave or oven and lay them on your tummy. They are very soothing!

Floradix and Liquid Chlorophyll are two supplements I like to use to keep my iron levels up and help my body replenish what it lost. They both help speed up the healing process and feed your body much needed minerals.

A Sitz bath really helps heal the area, especially if you tore. In His Hands carries several good options. They are very comforting and soothing to a new mama.

209

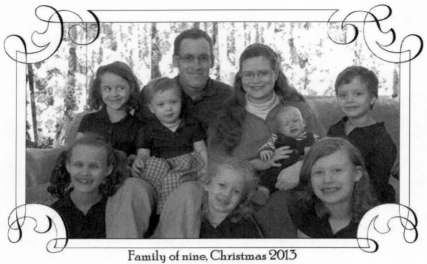

Family of nine, Christmas 2013

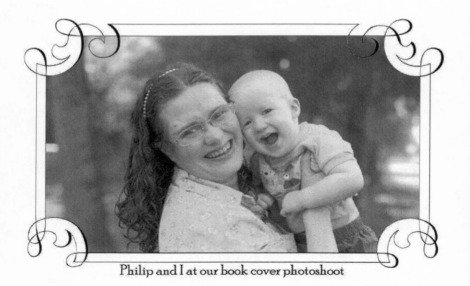

Philip and I at our book cover photoshoot

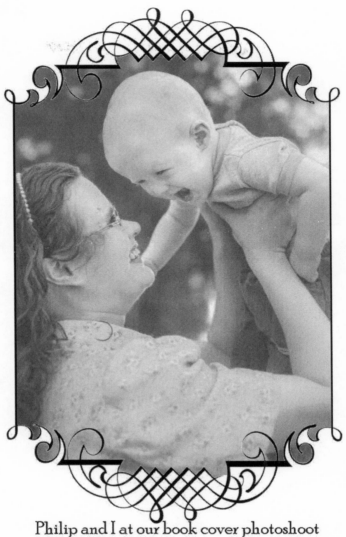

Philip and I at our book cover photoshoot

Epilogue

July 4, 2014

I was nearing the finalization of the first draft of this book. Philip was just a little guy still, so the memories were fresh.

"I'd better hurry and get this done before I get pregnant again," I told Nathan.

We talked about what we would do if I did get pregnant before I finished. Would I wait until I had the baby and write an extra chapter? Or would I not even mention it?

Well, this epilogue is the answer to that question! Yesterday, I got a positive test!!! I am pregnant with number 8. This is the first time I have ever gotten pregnant without having had a cycle, so our dates are a little sketchy. The best we can figure, I am likely due around the end of February.

You can get updates about this pregnancy on my blog. My website is **www.mistymarr.com**. You can also follow me on Facebook at:
www.facebook.com/mylessonslearned

September 3, 2014

Publication date is fast approaching, and anticipation is building as we finalize all the little details and final editing that goes along with publishing a book. What a journey this book experience has been!

I am hitting my second trimester. I've gone through the first trimester exhaustion, falling asleep while working on edit correction, and all that goes with that. I have weathered the worst of morning sickness, and an end is finally in sight!

I have struggled with some Lyme Disease setbacks, but nothing more than I should expect with pregnancy. My body has to switch from recovery mode to baby-making mode. I consider it a sacrifice worth making for the life of this new little one.

Yet, through it all, this book pushes ahead! I am glad to be able to share my story with you and to give God the glory for the good things He has done.

Nathan's Appendix

"Why Didn't You Limit Your Family Size?"

a theological framework for understanding our decisions

You have read in the preceding pages an account of many things that God has done in our family's life. I am sure that you have rejoiced with us in our good times and wept with us in the painful times. Perhaps some of you have asked very important and probing questions like, "Why would you put yourselves through so much pain and sorrow?" and "There are so many good birth control options available today. Why continue having children that cost you so much pain and difficulty?"

To be honest, we too have asked ourselves the same questions and there were times that we did not respond to these questions in faith but, rather, in doubt and fear. There were times in which we were like the disciple Peter (Matt 14:22-33) when he walked on the water to meet the Lord. As he focused on the wind and waves, his trust faltered and he began to sink. At times our faith has been shaken as well. In His mercy, God has reminded us of our own weakness and of our ongoing need for His help. His grace has been magnified in our weakness.

So why have we continued to have children even though it has cost us so much?

1. God made procreation to be one of the primary and foundational purposes for the family. In Genesis 1:27, God gives a mission statement to the family by saying, "Be fruitful and multiply and fill the earth and subdue it." We have continued to have children because it is an important part of God's purpose for the family. If we were to cut off that ability, we would disregard a significant portion of God's revealed will for our family's existence.

2. The gospel requires us to surrender our own life, take up our cross, and follow Christ (Matthew 16:24-25). To be a follower of Christ demands that the disciple "deny himself and take up his cross." Denial of self is giving up that which we naturally value: our comforts, our conveniences, and perhaps even our physical lives. In its original role, the cross was not a nice decoration or cultural symbol, but an instrument of death. Jesus calls us to take up the very instrument of our own demise and walk with him. He says that the contrast to the attitude of the disciple is a desire to save our own lives--desire for self-preservation. Mary, the mother of Jesus, was confronted with great loss when the angel Gabriel told her God's purpose for her life: to bring our Lord into this world in an unprecedented manner. For her, it

was a watershed moment. Would she take up her cross and follow or would she give in to the instinct of self-preservation and reject the plan. Her response was a statement of resolve that rings down through the centuries: "Behold, I am the servant of the Lord; let it be to me according to your word" (Luke 1:38, ESV). There is no equivocation in that statement. She is declaring her absolute commitment to God's plan, no loopholes no escape routes. She faced certain rejection and the probable loss of the opportunity to marry. In her way of thinking, this was doubtless a giving up of her life. This is the response of a disciple. We have continued to have children as an application of God's command to "be fruitful and multiply" because we desire to follow Christ as His disciples. Observant people have warned us that this practice of procreation could well be our destruction. This serves to remind me of the cross.

3. The discipleship that takes place in our home is an application of the Great Commission. We not only continue to have children because we are disciples but also because we desire to make disciples. We have many discipleship opportunities in life but none compare with the discipleship potential of a parent-child relationship. The impact of living life together and teaching them the commands of God--both through didactic instruction and sanctified example--is powerful. We desire to impact as many children as the Lord gives us. To purposefully limit the number of children we have

would be inconsistent with a commitment to follow the Great Commission.

4.   God places a very high value on children (Matthew 19:14; Luke 17:1-2). I presuppose that anything that God values is truly worthy of being valued. As Christians in the United States today, we have a choice: Will we emphasize those things that God values or the things that our culture says are valuable? A popular patriotic country song called "Chicken Fried" by the Zac Brown Band seeks to express our cultural ideals. I find this excerpt particularly descriptive of our values as a country:

I thank God for my life
And for the stars and stripes
May freedom forever fly, let it ring.
Salute the ones who died
The ones that give their lives
So we don't have to sacrifice
All the things we love

Like our chicken fried
And cold beer on a Friday night
A pair of jeans that fit just right
And the radio on

Our culture values stuff. Quality of living is our idol to such a degree that we "thank God" for other people who have given their lives to preserve our food, drink, clothes, and entertainment. I find the notion repulsive that someone would have to die so that I could eat fried chicken. We know that there are things worth giving our lives for, but fried chicken is not one of them. In contrast, God emphasizes the value of human life, and He teaches us that our life does not consist of the things that we possess. All the pretty things of this world are passing away (1 John 2:17), and even the most valuable and durable forms of wealth cannot be enjoyed for more than our short lifespan. But there is a real investment value to be had ... in the eternal souls of people. Parenting is a great investment opportunity.

5. God alone is the giver of life. I refuse to believe that x chromosome plus y chromosome equals an immortal soul. The life of a child in its mother's womb is the mysterious work of God (Ecclesiastes 11:5 Psalm 139:13-14). Sure, He uses the means of human participation but the Scriptures expressly say that God is the one who opens and closes the womb. In 1 Samuel 1, it says that Hannah's womb had been closed by the Lord. In response to her prayer, God opened her womb and gave her children. In Genesis 30, Jacob recognized that God was the one who managed the womb when He said to his discontented wife, "Am I in the place of God, who has withheld from you the fruit of the womb?" In opposition to the popular notion of our day, we don't believe that procreation is merely a matter of "women's health" to be treated and managed and, more often than not, prevented and squelched. Rather, it is a sacred participation with God in the

fulfillment of His expressed will of multiplying mankind.

These little children (soon to be big children) are our friends. Through them God has given us ample opportunity to lay down our lives and so, in some imperfect way, portray the love that Christ has shown for us in laying down His own life for our redemption. We rejoice in this exciting race which God has set before us.

"But God doesn't call us to be comfortable. He calls us to trust Him so completely that we are unafraid to put ourselves in situations where we will be in trouble if he doesn't come through."

Francis Chan

My Dad's Perspective

The Loss of a Child

By Mike Richardson, Spring 2005

As I walked into the house, Pam excitedly said, "Come here, I have something to show you." She was smiling broadly as she showed me a positive pregnancy test. God had chosen to bless us with another child—our tenth.

As the weeks passed, everyone became more and more excited. We talked about little boys and little girls. The topic of twins even came up on several occasions. Anna (7) said, "If you have twins, that will make eleven children; then if you have one more that will be twelve. Twelve is a good number!"

It came as a shock when Pam miscarried our little baby, David Michael, yesterday morning. Our hearts are saddened.

Until a few years ago, the word miscarriage had held no personal meaning to me. Then my daughter, Misty, had multiple miscarriages. I had only known a few women who had "lost" a baby. Most of the time people acted as though nothing had happened. Following a miscarriage, mothers have been told, "You're young. You'll have other babies. Forget about it."

Every baby, no matter how tiny or large, is a real person to God. "For You have formed my inward parts; You have covered me in my mother's womb. I will praise You, for I am fearfully and wonderfully made; marvelous are Your works, and that my soul knows very well. My frame was not hidden from You, when I was made in secret, and skillfully wrought in the lowest parts of the earth. Your eyes saw my substance, being yet unformed. And in Your book they all were written, the days fashioned for me, when as yet there were none of them." (Psalm 139:13-16)

When we sat down to tell our other children, there were many tears. Some were overwhelmed with a crushing, breathtaking grief. They had wanted this baby. They had already grown to love him. They/we didn't want any other baby; we wanted this one! Forget? How could we forget? Why should we forget? This was--no, is--our baby. Our baby died and I refuse to hide my grief! Many will act as if this pregnancy didn't happen. Some will expect me to also. I will not! He was my child and I loved him!

Nearly every parent's worst fear is the loss of a child— even those whose babies who haven't been born yet. The pain and grief suffered by moms and dads who have lost babies to miscarriage is just as real as the grief of those who lose children later in life.

The pain of losing a child is the most horrific thing imaginable to a mother or father! Yet God does heal the brokenhearted. Just as I refuse to hide my grief, I refuse to do anything other than place my confidence in God-- my Creator, my Savior. He heals the brokenhearted and binds up their wounds (Psalm 147:3).

Mike Richardson, Misty's daddy, is the father of ten children whose ages range from 37 to 6. He is also a missionary, a pastor, an author, publishes the Spanish home school magazine, *El Hogar Educador*, publishes books, CDs, DVDs in Spanish for the family, and is a beloved conference speaker at many Latin American homeschool conferences.

Lyme Disease Information

I am sure that many of you will have questions concerning Lyme Disease. I will answer a few of them now, but I also want to let you know that I do plan to write about my experience. My second book will be titled, *Lessons Learned: My Journey through Lyme Disease*. I plan to give much more in-depth information about my experience and what I have learned along the way.

I have not yet begun writing the book, but my hope is to have it available within a year. I cannot make any promises, but that is my goal.

I highly recommend the book, *Beating Lyme Disease* by Dr. David Jernigan. He is the founder of Hansa, the clinic that was so beneficial to me. I would recommend this book to anyone and everyone with Lyme Disease, no matter what route of treatment you use. It will be beneficial whether you choose to go completely conventional, natural only or anywhere in between. You will not regret this purchase!

If you are interested in the clinic, you can read about it at www.hansacenter.com. They have a great introductory video, and you can request the New Patient Package to be emailed to you for even more information. I HIGHLY recommend The Hansa Center for anyone dealing with Lyme Disease or any chronic illness. If you do go, please let them know that Misty Marr recommended you!

LESSONS LEARNED

One of the most helpful things I have learned about Lyme Disease is that the Lyme bacteria is constantly going through a cycle—they reproduce, they die, more reproduction, more dead Lyme. The Lyme emits toxins as it dies. These toxins are one of the biggest causes of many of the Lyme symptoms.

Since learning this, I have been able to significantly reduce the symptoms using intense methods of detoxification. My main treatment is doing a detox bath or using the far infrared sauna every day. I have done one or both of these 5-7 times a week since the beginning of my treatment, and they make the difference in my ability to even walk. If I skip a day or two, I begin to stumble, pain levels increase significantly and my neurological symptoms flare. You can Google "Dr. Jernigan's detox bath recipe" for instructions. His book will include that recipe and so much more!

The 2nd main part of what I did is use essential oils. I use a variety of them most days, and when I don't, I can feel the feel the difference. They really make a difference in my brain fog and ability to think. They significantly reduced my pain, as well.

I will share some of my favorite options.

Pain Relief: Pain Away, Deep Relief and Aroma Siez

Neurological/Brain Support: Helichrysum, Brain Power, Clarity, En-Er-Gee, Common Sense, Peppermint

Lyme Bug: Inner Defense, Lyme Bullet (uses Frankincense, Thieves and Oregano - Google for directions.)

Lyme Damage: Frankincense, Raindrop Treatment, Trauma Life, Valor

Sleep: Peace and Calming, Lavender, Rutavela and Sleep Essence

I use Ningxia Red to help keep my immune system strong and able to fight the lyme better. I use all of the above oils regularly, plus more. They are well worth the expense, as they make such a big difference in my ability to function.

I used the oils undiluted. I rub them on the bottom of my feet, my forehead, back of neck, temples, lymph nodes, back or wherever strikes my fancy. I also use them in a diffuser. Young Living oils are therapeutic grade and the ones listed as supplements can be ingested. I take the lyme bullet by mouth, at least. Most of the other's I use topically.

Many people sign up with Young Living as a distributor just for the discount, but others have found it to be a very profitable home business. You can order or enroll at **www.youngliving.com**. Please use my Distributor ID **1207823** in both the spots for Enroller and Sponsor ID's.

Please follow my website (www.mistymarr.com) or Facebook page (www.facebook.com/mylessonslearned) for more information and updates about Lessons Learned: My Journey through Lyme Disease. Meanwhile, the above suggestions can really help.

God bless you on your journey toward recovery!

Misty's Other Endeavors

In this section you will find a smorgasbord of products. For the record, I will personally benefit financially if you purchase through these links. Some are simply products that I receive commission from, others can be great home-business ideas for you as well. I appreciate your support as you help me provide for our family's needs! You can find direct links to these sites, plus a few more, on my website: **www.mistymarr.com**.

Lilla Rose

The Lilla Rose product line centers around unique, functional, and well-made hair jewelry. The Flexi clip will provide stylish ease for your everyday use, yet is elegant enough for the fanciest of hairdos. Not only is it feminine and stylish, it is practical and super easy to use. It is also very high quality. The Flexi Clip can be used to create multiple hair styles, and will work with all hair types. It will make moms feel attractive and allow them to keep their daughter's hair up with minimal effort, and is great for young ladies. Lilla Rose also has other high quality items such as bobby pins, headbands, hair sticks and more.

These are not only great for personal use, they make great gifts. Lilla Rose is also one of the best home business I have been involved it. Contact me through my Lilla Rose website for more information. **www.lillarose.biz/sweethairlooms**

Young Living

Young Living Essential oils have played a key role in my healing. I don't know how I would survive without them! They have a wide variety of therapeutic grade essential oils, plus a myriad of other health supplements. I highly recommend these oils! I use them daily. Many people sign up as a distributor just for the discount, but others have found it to be a very profitable home business. You can order or enroll at **www.youngliving.com**. Please use my ID **1207823** in both the spots for Enroller and Sponsor IDs.

Vitamix

The Vitamix is my all-time favorite kitchen appliance. I use it every day, often multiple times a day. It is so much more than just a blender. I often call it a blender on steroids. It is so powerful that it can blend a green smoothie to smooth perfection. It makes amazing frozen ice creams, can handle peanut butter, and so many other hard tasks. If you leave it on a little longer, it will heat, and boil your ingredients, allowing you to make a bowl of soup, a batch of pudding, or even a nice gravy without even turning on your stove. No stirring needed. The uses go on and on!